KV-702-486

OUR HEALTH, OUR LIVES

What women should know

Dr Susan R. Davis

ALLEN & UNWIN

613.042444. DAV.

UNIVERSITY OF LIMERICK
LIBRARY

01006249.

Copyright © Susan R. Davis, 1997

The information contained in this book is intended to be a guide for women. Neither Dr Susan Davis nor the Publisher can accept responsibility for your health or any side effects of the treatments outlined in this book. You should always consult your own doctor before following any treatment, whether it be conventional or natural therapy.

All rights reserved. No part of this book may be reproduced or transmitted in any form or by any means, electronic or mechanical, including photocopying, recording or by any information storage and retrieval system, without prior permission in writing from the publisher.

First published in 1997 by
Allen & Unwin Pty Ltd
9 Atchison Street, St Leonards NSW 2065 Australia
Phone: (61 2) 9901 4088
Fax: (61 2) 9906 2218
E-mail: frontdesk@allun-unwin.com.au
URL:http://www.allen-unwin.com.au

National Library of Australia
Cataloguing-in-Publication entry:

Davis, Susan (Susan Ruth), 1957– .
Our health, our lives: what women should know.

Includes index.
ISBN 1 86448 299 0.

1. Women—Health and hygiene. I. Title.

613.04244

Set in 12/14 pt Adobe Garamond by DOCUPRO, Sydney
Printed by Australian Print Group, Maryborough, Vic.

10 9 8 7 6 5 4 3 2 1

This book is dedicated to my four wonderful children, without whose love it could not have been written.

CONTENTS

INTRODUCTION

In the course of my work dealing with hormonal problems in women and female reproductive health, I regularly confront most of the health issues which trouble women. My patients and women friends are constantly asking me to recommend either specific or general reading material, but I have found that there is little published which fully answers their questions concerning many of the important women's health issues, especially in terms of disease prevention. Thus I have written this book as a comprehensive response to the questions regularly asked of me and the information sought by the women of varied ages and needs whom I encounter daily. My major emphasis, therefore, is on what women can do for themselves in terms of optimising health and well-being and disease prevention. I have purposely targeted health topics which are common, have major health consequences, are somewhat controversial and, I believe incompletely dealt with elsewhere.

It is my experience that women concerned about or suffering health disorders want to know as much as possible about their specific condition or interest, and so I make no apology for the depth of my discussion or the technical details in these pages. We can only make responsible health choices if fully aware of the facts, and it is facts that I have endeavoured to present in a clear and logical format.

I feel strongly that health is the responsibility of each individual. We all have to make lifestyle choices which impact on our own health and that of our families. Women are mostly the key decision-makers in the family unit and certainly set the family scene in terms of lifestyle. They are also the main educators in the family with respect to basics such as nutrition and sex education, as well as more abstract concepts such as self-esteem and body image. A woman needs to have a foundation of accurate information in aspects of basic health in order to teach the basics to her family. However, it is only possible for a woman to teach her children positive self-image and self-esteem if she feels confident and good about herself. It is my intention that the contents of this book will assist women with both the tangible and the abstract concepts of good health.

There are obviously many medical conditions and disease states that are unique to women. However, it is being increasingly recognised that several diseases common to both sexes, such as cardiovascular disease and diabetes, affect women differently from men. I have therefore described the various ways in which patterns of disease in women differ from men and I have focused on the preventive strategies and aspects of treatment that are specific to women.

The controversies in women's health are not always immediately apparent. I have tried to increase the awareness of debate in several areas such as natural therapies and breast cancer, and provide the facts that are to hand. I chose not to provide references as I felt they would detract from the readability of the text, although I am aware that some readers would prefer that specific references be included. All the information in this book is based on published medical literature, apart from where I have specifically stated that something is my personal opinion or belief, and much of what I have written here has been the subject of work I have written and published in various international, refereed medical journals. Many aspects of preventive health which I have discussed, particularly in the chapters on body image and body weight and cardiovascular disease, are equally applicable to men and I believe preventive health in men should be a high community priority. However, I have specifically written this book for a female readership and consequently I have focused on the health problems faced by women.

In conclusion, I can only hope that I have achieved what I set out to do, and that everyone who reads part or all of this book will benefit in some way.

BEING IN CONTROL

Most women want to enjoy their lives and consider any health problem a nuisance, not a focus. They do not choose to be unwell. By virtue of their reproductive status, however, women from a young age are subject to a variety of troublesome symptoms which interfere with their quality of life and necessitate their consulting the medical profession. Their health problems range from menstrual disorders through to concerns about body hair, sexuality, fertility and, from the start of sexual activity, cancer prevention and detection. Frequently, women feel their problems are not severe enough to warrant seeking medical advice. For example, at what level of discomfort or pain should a young woman seek help for monthly menstrual cramps? Too many women have felt trivialised in the past when told their symptoms are minor, or due to stress, or something they must learn to live with. Such experiences resulted in women putting up with symptoms unnecessarily. These symptoms may be a manifestation of an underlying stressful life situation or psychological problems; more commonly, however, they have a biological cause, although sometimes they are exacerbated by psychological factors. Health professionals should be able to help women gain insight into the physical, psychological and social factors modifying or aggravating their symptoms and direct them towards learning how to deal with health problems as they arise. Women need the opportunity and adequate time to discuss their health problems and learn about preventive health practices. All women should feel that their health concerns are dealt with in context with their own health expectations which means that every woman needs to be treated as an individual.

Health needs vary with the stages of life. Our quality of life depends not only on good health but also on our environment, social circumstances and cultural expectations. Women need to be wary of comparing their own health needs and treatment to those of others. For example, it is common for women to sit and chat about childbirth, comparing their experiences, whether their childbirth was 'natural' or whether pain relief such as pethidine or an epidural were administered. But no two experiences of childbirth are ever the same or comparable, even the different pregnancies of the same woman. No one except the woman involved can experience the pain and decide what she needs. Similarly, menstrual pain or migraine or menopausal symptoms are unique personal experiences. No one has the right to discourage or deny other women relief from their symptoms on the basis that these are all natural reproductive phenomena. It is just as reasonable for older women to take oestrogen to eliminate distressing menopausal hot flushes as it is for younger women to take anti-inflammatory medicine to relieve menstrual pain.

USING HEALTH SERVICES

Every woman has the right to maximise her own quality of life by taking steps to optimise her own health. Health information should be available so that each woman can make her own choice about relevant health issues. This requires women to take responsibility for their own health as users of health services or as patients. For example, it is difficult to have a comprehensive medical consultation while dealing with bored or distressed children. When attending their doctor, women with young children should plan ahead when possible and organise some form of childcare so they can focus on themselves for a few minutes and allow the doctor to interact with them on a one-to-one basis. Thinking ahead about what is expected from the consultation can be extremely helpful. Is the doctor being seen for advice, for symptoms which require diagnosis and management, for a specific investigation, such as a Pap smear, or for treatment, such as contraception? It can be useful to make a list of all the symptoms or problems to be discussed before the consultation—it's easy to forget even important things. This list need only be brief. Too much detail will only blur the major issues. It is also appropriate to ask why certain blood tests or X-rays or other investigations need to be performed and whether any risk is involved. In addition, it is wise to ask about the meaning of the diagnosis and any future implications and request that the doctor writes down the name of the suspected or diagnosed conditions.

Responsibility entails knowing the name, not just the colour, of any prescribed medication and asking about possible side-effects. If drug treatment is chosen, each woman should discuss how long she wants to take the medication before stopping it and reassessing the need to continue. It is always important to have a treatment plan at the commencement of any therapy so that the treatment goals and the way in which the outcome of treatment is to be assessed is clear for both the doctor and the patient.

It is always good to question whether there are any other ways of dealing with a specific condition. For example, high cholesterol can be treated with medication but this should be seen as a last resort by both parties. Ideally, lifestyle modifications involving dietary changes and a formal exercise program should be the first step to lowering cholesterol. The latter is the more difficult treatment path, because it requires patient involvement and commitment. In this formula, the doctor acts as the educator and prescriber of good health practices and the patient takes an active rather than passive role in her own health management. This is how it should be. Your health is your responsibility.

LIFE PLANNING

Good health doesn't come in a magic pill. It requires a lifetime plan, involving several key factors: a healthy diet, physical activity, avoiding or minimising the intake of deleterious substances (alcohol, caffeine, drugs and tobacco) and, most importantly, psychological well-being. So many diseases plaguing Western society are preventable. For example, lung cancer has overtaken breast cancer as the leading cause of cancer death in women in the United States. This reflects the increasing number of women smoking. Most of these cancer deaths would be prevented by women not smoking. Bowel cancer is almost unheard of in traditional African communities where a low fat, high fibre diet is the norm. It is the third most common cancer in women in the Western world, again due to poor diet. The link between prolonged exposure to the sun and skin cancer is well known, especially in Australia where the rate of melanoma is the highest in the world. Sensible sun protection by using sunscreens and hats will prevent most skin cancers. The feature common to these cancers and many other diseases is that they are easily prevented.

Consideration to the health consequences of lifestyle, having normal body weight, being physically active and eating well are unquestionably the keys to good health. Although the formula sounds simple, it's not always so with the lifestyle pressures of the 1990s. But taking responsibility for your health is truly worth the effort.

PSYCHOLOGICAL WELL-BEING

Psychological health and well-being is inseparable from physical health. Our psychological state influences our physical capacity and body functions. We have all had the experience of being anxious or nervous and having 'butterflies in the stomach'. This is a classic example of a physical response to a psychological stress. People who are chronically stressed frequently feel excessively tired or suffer headaches or experience other physical symptoms. Stress, depression and low self-esteem make us more physically vulnerable and aggravate all disease processes.

Important brain centres which are affected by stress and mood interact with the immune system, the body's defence against infections and cancer. Excessive stress depresses the immune system and increases the risk of developing ill health. The stress may be psychological or physical. Some examples of the former would be chronic work stress, financial stress or emotional stress, such as loss of a loved one. Physical stress can take the form of a major illness, but also includes chronic, extreme physical exertion as endured by elite athletes, long-distance runners providing the classic example. Long-term overexercising and chronic psychological stress have been found to cause depression of the immune system. Reducing stress takes the pressure off the immune system and allows the body's defences to get on with their job—hence the success of meditation and relaxation programs as adjuncts to cancer therapy.

Women are more likely to experience ill health and report more symptoms of menstrual disturbances or menopausal symptoms if they are experiencing major life stress, are depressed, or have low self-esteem. Poor self-esteem does not in itself cause ill health, but it can be considered another form of psychological stress which makes us more vulnerable to diseases and the effects of ill health. Stress and depression lower the threshold for discomfort or pain, and many other symptoms like headaches, migraines or back pain are amplified when we are psychologically compromised. In such situations, we feel less in control of our bodies, and our symptoms take over. It becomes more difficult to act positively to alleviate the discomfort and in turn we are less able to cope.

So irrespective of age or gender, identifying and then minimising stress and developing and maintaining good psychological health are crucial to good general health, the end point of which is quality and enjoyment of life. Really, that's what it's all about.

Several wonderful self-help books which specifically deal with topics ranging from meditation and relaxation through to assertiveness, self-knowledge and improving self-esteem are widely available and are found by many people to be very useful. Similarly there are many personal development courses run by recognised community adult education groups which address these issues, and are highly recommended.

The path to good health resides not only in taking responsibility for ourselves but also in listening to and nurturing our bodies. One of the fundamental principles of the natural therapies is to teach people to nurture, support and respect their own bodies, all things many women put at the bottom of the priority list. These things mean allowing time to care for ourselves and being aware of our personal needs.

We all have individual body rhythms and those of us who are tuned into their own biorhythms cope much better. For example, many important hormones in the body are produced and released in a specific 24-hour cyclic pattern. These are called *circadian rhythms*. They affect different people in different ways. Some of us feel better and more energetic in the morning whereas others have energy surges at other times of the day. If you recognise when you feel best then you can use that time most productively. Women with menstrual problems can use pattern recognition to identify times of peak symptoms and then deal specifically with the symptoms when they are anticipated. For example, a woman may avoid stressful work situations when she is aware that she is premenstrual. Alternatively, she may recognise that she is feeling irritable and anxious premenstrually and deal more effectively with stressful situations at that time because of the awareness of her own responses and reactions.

Positive action with respect to our health involves a whole range of lifelong preventive health measures. Women during their reproductive years need to have regular medical screens for cervical cancer (Pap smear tests) and breast cancer (mammography). It is important to develop a relationship with a family doctor with whom you feel comfortable, who can provide preventive health advice and perform or arrange the required health screening procedures.

OUR HEALTH, OUR LIVES: KNOWLEDGE AND RESPONSIBILITY

Find out as much as you can about your own body. Women in general, and adolescents in particular, still don't know enough about their bodies. There are many aspects of health which have been extensively featured in the media, but the available information is frequently both conflicting and confusing. One study which addressed the beliefs and feelings of Australian girls about menstruation found that their knowledge was very limited, and mixed up with many incorrect and negative myths. Overall, they expressed embarrassment and ambivalence about menstruating and had developed varying coping strategies including denial and self-deception. The information may be out there but it is still not getting through to the young girls who need it in simplified but comprehensive terms. Clearly health education programs need to specifically target prepubescent children and negative attitudes and myths about topics like menstruation need to be dispelled. The greater the understanding women of all ages have about the function and responses of their own bodies, the more likely they are to be able to care properly for themselves and be proud of and enjoy their bodies.

Heart disease, diabetes, bowel cancer, lung cancer, skin cancer, and most probably breast and prostate cancer, are the end result of the interaction between genetics, lifestyle, poor eating patterns and the changing late twentieth century environment. It's ironic that with our advanced medical technology and knowledge these diseases not only exist but are on the increase. Science and technology cannot cure the fundamental negative Western lifestyle factors that are contributing to ill health. There is no medicine that can counteract a sedentary lifestyle, chronic stress, alcohol consumption, cigarette smoking or a high fat, calorie dense diet. From an early age we are exposed to the pressure of living and as a result of technology we are now able to and expect to pack more into each day than ever before. The detrimental health aspects of what is considered to be a normal lifestyle affect men and women equally, but the greatest impact is on the most recent generation which is demonstrating higher rates of obesity, diabetes and other lifestyle-related illnesses. Being aware of and understanding what is basically healthy and unhealthy at the level of day-to-day living is the first step towards better health and disease prevention for both the individual and the community. The following chapters address some important women's health issues including body image and weight, menstrual disorders, excess body hair, natural therapies, premature menopause, breast cancer, cardiovascular disease and sexuality. The emphasis is on the causes of ill health and ways in which changes in lifestyle can improve health and hopefully enhance the quality of life. The contents are by no means definitive but are intended to be informative, stimulating and provocative, and to extend the basis upon which we as women can build up our knowledge about ourselves and our bodies and thus be more in control of our health and our lives.

2

BODY IMAGE AND BODY WEIGHT

It's great to feel healthy and feel that you look good. In fact, there is nothing wrong with wanting to look good. Controversy exists, however, over the definition of 'looking good', the extremes to which some individuals go in order to achieve the desired 'look' and the low self-esteem so many suffer because their body image—that is, their perception of how they appear to others—doesn't match their expectations.

Enjoying a healthy lifestyle means having an appropriate diet, sufficient pleasurable exercise and satisfaction with your place in society. When any of these ingredients in the feel-good-about-yourself recipe fails, then self-esteem is at risk. Dissatisfaction with where we are 'at' in life can be enough to distort body image—even when we look wonderful to others. An example of this would be the healthy adolescent, who, despite appearing physically attractive to others, develops a distorted body image (that she is too fat), as a result of feelings of inadequacy, and diets madly, ultimately spiralling into a state of anorexia nervosa.

The big question is why do the majority of women in the Western world have so much difficulty with their body image and appearance?

BEAUTY AND THINNESS

Beauty is culturally defined. The current concept of female beauty in twentieth century Western society is very different from the voluptuous, pear-shaped female physique which had been accepted by women and celebrated in art through the ages. The socio-cultural physical ideal for affluent women in Western society now is thinness. A study of *Playboy* centre-folds and Miss America winners over the 25 years up until 1980 found the young women featured had progressive reductions in waist and hip measurements and body weight. In complete contrast, the general American population has become heavier. Many experts writing in the area believe that male-domination of our society is to blame for the female quest for thinness. Interestingly, the desire for a thin, android body shape has only emerged in the last 30 or so years after centuries of male-domination. Many men still prefer women to be fleshier and bustier than women themselves would choose to be. If anything, the emergence of the thinness fad paralleled the sexual revolution of the 1960s and appears to be more an expression of women taking control over their own bodies and choosing how they want to look and dress, rather than allowing their concept of beauty to be dictated to them by men.

In 1960 the American Food and Drug Administration approved the sale of Enovid, the first publicly available oral contraceptive pill. This new method of birth control opened the floodgates of the sexual revolution. Women suddenly had access to control over their reproductive capacity enabling sexual experimentation. Over the ensuing years societal, especially female, expectations of female sexuality, broadened with an acceptance of the right for women to manifest their sexual curiosity and express their sexuality. This was reflected in the dramatic change in the way women began to dress in the 1960s and 1970s, compared to the 1950s and earlier.

Feminist philosophy of the 1970s proclaimed that the overwhelming desire of young girls and women to be 'beautiful' is driven by the male domination of female sexuality and the manipulation of the female psyche and attitudes towards beauty by men. Earlier, Simone de Beauvoir had proposed that women mostly visualise themselves as men define them, not in accordance with their normal innate selves. It was said that the male had stolen the female body.

These were certainly valid concepts historically and still apply to many women in various cultures today. Having experienced sexual liberation, however, Westernised women have themselves redefined the 'ideal' female physique in the context of their new sexual freedom. *Women* have taken control over their expectations of female beauty in recent years, and the endemic pursuit of thinness is no longer dominated by men but is largely generated and perpetuated by women. Adolescent girls are now more conscious of their sexuality than in the past. This is reflected in the prevailing female fashion, which is not only perhaps more provocative than ever before but also generally accepted by Western communities. Bare midriffs and scanty tops that cannot be differentiated from undergarments are common clothing choices of young women who are enjoying a degree of physical freedom. Being thin, even waif-like, is also part of this fashion trend. Popular music and music video clips which are important in the establishment of trends in dressing and other aspects of appearance, have been criticised for familiarising adolescents with a broad spectrum of female sexuality and sex appeal. Certainly this exposure at such a young age is unprecedented, but this form of media is not necessarily bad. Many of the music video clips of female pop icons present these women in a very positive manner in that they appear assertive, independent and are often depicted in positions of power, and their provocative dressing and thin physiques are mostly associated with strong female independence, not male domination.

The societal concept or definition of the body beautiful must be separated from the current preoccupation of Western society to achieve beauty and the overvaluing of beauty to the point that physical attractiveness is equated with success. This issue affects both men and women.

The 1960s and 1970s resulted in increased freedom of sexual expression for men as well as women. Coincident with this was the increasing public awareness of diet and exercise for good health and then, during the 1980s, the cultural value of thinness increased. Pritikin blazed the fat free, low cholesterol, jogging trail and subsequently society has come to favour the lean, athletic look. This shift in the concept of beauty occurred during the economic boom of the 1980s, during which time Western society became incredibly achievement-oriented with individuals succumbing to extraordinarily high self-expectations. Not only did people want to 'make it' but doing so required looking good too. Some considered thinness and beauty more important female attributes than intelligence for women to succeed, especially some women. This overemphasis on appearances, however, has not been restricted to women but many men have felt the same pressure to achieve the desired athletic, firm appearance in order to fit the socially desired setting. Slimness has become a mark of success and control. Sub-populations have emerged within which slimness is an especially important norm. The emphasis is on acceptability, achievement and control. It is my view that the preoccupation with the way we look, particularly thinness, is a pathological manifestation of dysfunctional Western culture as a whole. It is a disease of affluence and consumerism. Non-affluent societies cannot afford the luxury of this overwhelming desire, commonly combined with great effort, to achieve the lean look. The body build in terms of fatness of people in developing nations is dictated by their lifestyle, including daily physical exertion and the availability of food. They don't have to work at being thin, it is intrinsic to their existence. In contrast, people in some industrialised countries overly focus on being thin, not usually in the context of being healthy but by relating thinness with beauty. The media and the advertising machine, again driven by economics, continue to reinforce the individual's wish to achieve beauty, irrespective of gender. This is intricately bound up with the enormous pressure on individuals to achieve. Good body image is inseparable from personal identity and self-esteem. The pursuit of beauty, including thinness, is not just a female issue but a societal issue. Feminist authors and artists in the 1960s and 1970s worked towards enhancing the self-esteem of women and their regard for their own bodies and sexuality. Now society as a whole may need rescuing from the prevailing pressure on appearances.

ATTITUDES TOWARDS AGEING

Inseparable from the body image issue is the prevailing preoccupation with youth in Western society. The physical changes that accompany ageing are feared by men and women alike, so much so that the ageing process is considered repulsive, the aged are treated as socially illegitimate and to appear forever young is desirable. Older women often recount experiences of being made to feel 'invisible' in certain social situations as their aged appearance and presence doesn't seem appropriate, or that younger people don't even look at them, but look through them. Age is associated with social isolation, loneliness, and as one woman put it, 'the loss of personhood'. Many people who are concerned that having physical features associated with ageing, such as greying hair and wrinkling, feel they must do everything in their power to combat these changes in order to retain their social acceptability. Much of the cosmetic industry—and in this I also include some forms of cosmetic surgery, beauty therapies and health centres rely on the public paranoia of this inevitable ageing process. Ageing should be acknowledged with dignity and respect. We seem to have forgotten the positive and desirable aspects of ageing: that perspective and wisdom require the combination of long experience and an ability to stand back a little from the chaos of life, attributes which usually only develop with advancing age. We need to reflect upon the modern Western attitude towards ageing in comparison to the way in which more traditional cultures deal with this life phase. People of advanced age in Asian cultures are treated with respect, their contributions to family and society are valued and are considered to be essential for a stable, functional community. Considering the increasing proportion of older people in Western cultures, our attitudes toward ageing require a great deal of reconsideration.

WHAT IS DESIRABLE IN TERMS OF BODY WEIGHT?

The odd thing about this whole issue is that despite the fact that being thin, athletic and youthful is considered almost synonymous with beauty and 'goodness', and that extensive public health education programs addressing diet and exercise have been running for years, the populations of the industrialised countries are progressively getting fatter and unhealthier. There appears to be a divergence in society so that some individuals, usually those with high self-expectations, respond to the cultural pressure towards slimness by focusing on diet, exercise and weight control, whereas others respond to the abundance and availability of food with resultant weight excess. Virtually all eating disorders, ranging from anorexia nervosa through to extreme obesity, are diseases of affluence. In the eighteenth and nineteenth centuries, when food was basic and often scarce, weight was equated with wealth and eating disorders were rare. In this century, most industrial countries have been freed of the fear of outright starvation. People are no longer concerned whether they are able to obtain enough food to survive but rather how to deal with the choice of food with which they are confronted. This is a bizarre luxury unique to the twentieth century.

Although the idealisation and pursuit of thinness is highlighted in the media, the health hazards that result from being overweight are a greater burden to the community. In this context the maintenance of normal body weight is a health issue not an aesthetic one. Excessive weight leads to increased heart disease, diabetes, cancer risk and joint problems, and the list goes on. The concept of excess weight is not simple. Women genetically tend to carry fat around their hips, bottoms and thighs and are said to have a *gynoid* body shape. This is not weight excess but hormonally appropriate fat storage. Fat in the lower third of the body is not associated with disease. In contrast, fat stored centrally and in the upper body is strongly associated with diseases such as diabetes, high blood pressure, high cholesterol and atherosclerosis. From a health perspective, a spare tyre or two around the middle is undesirable, but padding around the hips and thighs is just fine. So to be healthy, we don't need to be ultra lean, or have a figure like a model. (The impact of having too much central body fat on health is addressed in Chapter 8.)

OBESITY, AN EMERGING ISSUE

In countries like the United States and Australia, being overweight is becoming progressively more socially acceptable. For example, in the US, overweight women are recognised as an increasingly important consumer group by the clothing industry. In response to consumer demand, the major up-market stores are expanding their departments of designer label clothing for sizes 18 and above. Big-size fashion is currently the most rapidly growing area of the American clothing industry in terms of sales and profits, reflecting the community's increasing acceptance of obesity.

The problem of obesity is emerging in Asian and some African countries, which are becoming progressively industrialised and urbanised. In Asia, people in rural communities have a lower average body weight than urban dwellers, although the average body weight adjusted for height is still less than that of inhabitants of developed countries. Greater body weight and obesity is associated with indices of affluence, namely higher education, greater income and higher occupational status. Increased weight in Asian communities is also correlated with high blood cholesterol and blood pressure. These changes reflect the trends towards a more Western-style diet. Diseases such as diabetes and coronary artery disease, which were once rare among black South Africans, are now common causes of morbidity and death in the urbanised black community. The major factors leading to such illnesses are the increased consumption of poor quality, calorie dense foods and a more sedentary lifestyle, accompanied again with an increasing community acceptance of obesity.

Obesity is both an individual and a community issue in terms of general attitudes towards food and eating patterns. Many women's social lives, either within or beyond the home, revolve around food. Food is not only abundant, but also a domestic and communal focus. It represents giving, sharing, loving and celebrating. People eat in a socially dictated pattern, rarely as a response to their individual biological needs. Studies have shown that the dietary intake of sedentary people is poorly linked to their energy needs, whereas active people are more likely to consume an amount of food that matches their energy requirements. In conflict with the excessive cultural value placed on slimness, there is concurrently an inappropriate value placed on food. Food is big business. Consumers are prey to elaborate advertising designed to persuade them to indulge in specific food products. Food items are modified to have maximum appeal in terms of look and taste as well as ease of preparation. Fast food, junk food (concentrated sugars and fats) and instant food are all inexpensive and readily available. People now have to 'control' their food consumption. This isn't how it's meant to be—we should have food to live, not live for food. Jill Dupleix in her wonderful book *New Food* (William Heinemann, Melbourne, 1994) comments, 'It's time we changed the way we eat . . . We have the chance to learn from the past to safeguard our future, and to adjust our eating so that we eat better and feel better every day.'

Just as we have developed a somewhat distorted image of what is beautiful in terms of human aesthetics, we have also developed a distorted concept of the quantity and type of food we need to eat. Most people simply overeat, but are unaware that they are doing so since food has become so accessible and our social norms regarding the appropriate intake of food have increased. Over the years food has become more palatable and huge amounts of calories are consumed in concentrated forms as sweets and fats. Food is no longer for sustenance alone, but a taste experience and as much emphasis is placed on its appearance and novelty as on its taste. We have become a 'McDonalds society', expecting and enjoying fast food and instant gratification.

There are large numbers of people who have dieted for many years and still fail to lose weight. Their metabolism appears to partially shut down as they semi-starve themselves, and the anticipated weight loss doesn't eventuate. It is well established that extreme diets do not work. In order to lose weight we need to eat enough to fuel the system and switch the body's metabolism on, combined with sufficient activity to burn up excess energy.

Furthermore, much attention has recently become focused on genetic predisposition to obesity. The mouse obesity (ob) gene and its human equivalent have now been identified and cloned. The product of the ob gene is a protein called *leptin*, from the Greek word 'leptos' which means thin. This particular protein circulates in the blood of mice and humans, and appears to induce an unconscious reduction in food intake and enhanced physical activity resulting in weight loss. A particular strain of mice appears to be resistant to the actions of this protein and thus overeat and become obese. Similarly, obese humans have been found to have high blood levels of leptin, up to five times higher than non-obese people, and also appear to be resistant to its biological actions. It is believed that sensitivity to leptin may also be important in diet-induced obesity, in which severe dieting is followed by a rebound increase in body weight. However, for the majority of people the old-fashioned adage still holds true: you are what you eat.

If you consume more energy than you need then your balance is positive and you gain weight. To lose excess weight you must either eat less, (but not to an extreme) or exercise more, but ideally, do both.

WHAT CAN BE DONE?

Dealing with this issue requires a resetting of individual and community attitudes toward body weight and body image and food. First, you must view food simply as food. It can be attractive, but it should be good for you. Taste it, enjoy it, indulge yourself by eating better food from natural ingredients with more flavour. Don't diet. Just try to only eat *what* you need *when* you need it. It is often helpful to keep a food diary for a couple of days. This means writing down literally every item of food and drink that goes into your mouth. You don't need to add up the calories, but just look at how much and when you have eaten. Many people are shocked by the amount they inadvertently and unconsciously consume. Then go back to the beginning. Think about it once more. Listen to your body, it knows when and what you should eat. Reconsider your *attitude* toward food. Let it be a functional item over which *you* have total control—and don't let other people hassle you. Initially your friends will support and admire you for losing weight and then they'll envy you and maybe even resent your success! Women tell of friends who try to entice them with food to stop them achieving what they themselves have failed to do.

Next consider your activity level.

Sedentary people burn up energy slowly, whereas active individuals have a more rapid metabolism. Prioritise your life. Designate specific periods of time in your week when you can do some formal exercise. Generally women have the most difficulty doing this. They feel primarily obligated to their husbands, children, friends and work and this dictates how they spend their time. It's OK to be a little bit 'selfish' in order to create some time each week to devote to your health. Women who exercise feel better, have more energy, sleep better and generally are healthier in body and mind. Women must appreciate that by looking after their own health and well-being, they are indirectly looking after the health of their family and loved ones. So go for it! Don't be over-ambitious, there's no point in planning to do what you clearly cannot achieve. Begin gradually, exercising within your capacity for short periods and gradually increasing your exercise time. Make your exercise an integral part of your life, a time you can share with others. Walk or cycle with a friend, or join a swimming group at a local pool. Exercising with other people can be a great social extension for those who are otherwise socially isolated, and exercise has no age limit. Try to find a form of exercise you enjoy so it can be a pleasurable part of your life, not a punishment. And most importantly, stick with it: it will benefit your mind and your body.

OBESITY IN CHILDREN

Of great concern is the impact of dietary trends and lifestyle on the children and adolescents of the 1990s. Not only are adults becoming more overweight and less active but our children are also getting fatter and exercising less. Childhood obesity is no longer uncommon. In Australia, the average weight of twelve-year-old girls was three kilograms greater in 1994 than in 1985, and the average weight of fourteen-year-old boys has increased by six kilograms in the same time frame. Inherited genes are important determinants of obesity; however, environmental factors such as having a high fat, high calorie diet and a sedentary lifestyle also play a major role. Children are more likely to consume calorie dense, convenience food and engage in sedentary entertainment such as electronic games and home videos than their counterparts a decade ago. The hours commonly spent watching television significantly contribute to childhood obesity. Sitting in front of the television requires no energy apart from the basic amount necessary for the resting body. Plus, children's prime time television is the target of the sophisticated marketing of predominantly non-nutritious, calorie rich foods, which are in turn likely to be consumed by children watching increasing amounts of television. Time spent watching television detracts from time spent in energetic activity. Among twelve to seventeen-year-olds, the prevalence of obesity increases by two per cent for every additional hour of television watched. Many school-aged children do not participate in any form of regular sport, let alone kick a football in the street or ride their bicycles around the neighbourhood. This lessened physical activity affects not only the general health and well-being of children, but also their development of normal motor skills, like strength and co-ordination. We know that the development of fine motor skills such as writing or playing an instrument is dependent on having good gross motor skills (running, jumping, throwing etc.). Australian research tells us that less than 50 per cent of primary school children in Victoria can catch a ball properly. Of the twelve-year-olds studied, only about one-third could catch a ball and less than ten per cent could jump, run, bounce, throw or kick a ball at the level expected of a child aged six or seven. This is extremely worrying. At a very young age, many children have an established lifestyle pattern which is associated with considerable health problems if continued into adult life. We know that eating habits, and probably also exercise patterns, developed in childhood are likely to carry through into adult life. Death from all causes, but specifically from coronary heart disease, stroke and bowel cancer, is greater among those who have been overweight in adolescence than for those who were lean. The effect of being overweight in the teenage years on adult health may be due to the central body deposition of fat that occurs in adolescence, and to the early changes that can occur in the arteries of children which precede the development of atherosclerosis.

Women who have been overweight in adolescence are more likely to suffer arthritic problems in later years and have difficulty with activities of daily living such as walking and climbing stairs. Thus there are a number of adverse health effects which occur in adulthood that are associated with being overweight in the childhood and teenage years. So not only must we try to be active and eat well ourselves, but we must also teach our children how to eat properly and encourage their involvement in sports at school as well as other physical activities that ideally can involve the whole family. The emphasis, however, is on eating well and being physically active. It should not be on dieting and being thin. Children and adolescents must have sufficient energy for healthy growth and development. They need to be encouraged to choose nutritious food and to eat what they need, but not to focus on food inappropriately.

THE EATING DISORDERS: ANOREXIA NERVOSA AND BULIMIA

Anorexia nervosa is an illness characterised by extreme weight loss, distorted body image and the overriding fear of becoming obese. *Bulimia* is quite a different problem of secretive binge-eating and self-induced vomiting, with each episode

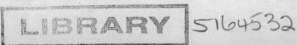
LIBRARY 5164532

being followed by bouts of guilt and shame and low self-esteem. Anorexia nervosa is a disorder which affects predominantly women (only one male for every nine females) whereas bulimia, which was originally believed to predominate in women, appears to also affect a large number of men. Extreme weight consciousness usually first appears in childhood, not during adolescence, although the actual eating disorder does not usually evolve until the teenage years. However, anorexia nervosa is not limited to young people and may affect people later in life. Over 70 per cent of young women in Northern Europe and North America believe they are overweight, even when their body weight is below normal or normal. Anorexia nervosa affects one out of every 100 girls in British secondary schools and up to twenty per cent of high school and university students have been reported as having some experience of bulimia. One study found that ten per cent of females interviewed at a suburban shopping centre had a lifetime history of bulimia.

Anorexia nervosa is unfortunately relatively common and its incidence has doubled over the last two decades. It may begin abruptly or develop insidiously. It tends to affect people at a younger age than bulimia, usually between the ages of twelve and the mid-thirties, whereas bulimia more commonly begins in the late teenage years. Both bulimia and anorexia are serious, potentially life-threatening conditions. The death rate from anorexia nervosa, excluding deaths from suicide, has been reported as being as high as nine per cent. Fundamentally death occurs as a result of extreme starvation. The long-term medical consequences of less severe forms of anorexia nervosa include oestrogen deficiency and osteoporosis, renal impairment from chronic dehydration and cardiovascular changes, including thinning of the heart muscle wall and altered heart function. Despite weight gain and apparent 'recovery' with return of normal menstruation, many sufferers of anorexia nervosa continue to have psychological problems which interfere with their lives.

A standard set of criteria for the diagnosis of anorexia nervosa and bulimia have been established. Cardinal features of anorexia nervosa include loss of more than 25 per cent of original body weight in conjunction with refusal to maintain normal body weight, disturbed body image and dread of becoming overweight. The diagnosis of bulimia is based on recurring episodes of excessive eating, terminated by vomiting, abdominal pain or sleep and followed by depression. The affected individual is aware of her disturbed eating pattern and frightened by her loss of control.

Many people demonstrate anorexic-like behaviour in that they are very obsessive about their food intake and weight, exercise intensely and have a perpetual fear of becoming fat, but this is not true anorexia nervosa. Similarly, some people are overweight and binge-eat, but do not go to the punitive extremes of bulimics.

Unfortunately it is not uncommon for sufferers of anorexia nervosa and their families to deny their illness, and to refuse medical and psychiatric care. Anorexia nervosa is a serious disorder and once identified should be treated by physicians experienced with this condition. Various therapies can be used, but initially it is imperative that the physical status and the risk of death of the affected individual is properly assessed. People with bulimia are more likely to seek out help and now there are self-help groups such as Eaters Anonymous, which offer wonderful support.

There are several theories as to why these disorders develop. Young women with anorexia and bulimia classically are high achievers, especially at school, who experience some stressful change at school or in their home or social environment. Depression and other eating disorders and alcoholism are not uncommon in the families of affected girls. Obesity in childhood is sometimes followed by severe dieting during the teenage years, accompanied by a preoccupation with food and ultimately the development of either anorexia or bulimia.

Other 'risk' families include those in which either siblings or parents have a weight problem, or in contrast, families in which fitness, sport and good eating are excessively emphasised or achievement-oriented families. Again, it all comes back to the cultural preoccupation equating appearances and slimness with achievement, control and fundamentally being loved. The various theories as to what finally precipitates an eating disorder including the following.

- *Psychological theory*. Control of eating is used as a defence against anxiety and psychosexual issues.
- *Social theory*. Eating disorders are precipitated by the emphasis on thinness in a male dominated society where a woman is loved for her appearance.
- *Family theory*. The affected individual is the identified patient in an 'ill family'. What this means is that the whole family has a problem or various problems, although most of the members of the family are able to continue to get by. The child with anorexia nervosa can be seen as the 'symptom' of the whole family being unwell. Her illness really reflects the problem that the entire family is suffering (but may not choose to acknowledge this). The continuation of this theory is that the girl with anorexia nervosa cannot be treated in isolation. Her entire family needs assessment and counselling in order for her to become well again.
- *Learning theory*. Unacceptable eating behaviour results in attention, therefore a good way to continue to get attention and have control over others is to continue the unacceptable eating pattern. For example, dinner on the table followed by refusal to eat results in attention from parents which then reinforces the behaviour.
- *Developmental theory*. Anorexia nervosa or bulimia develop as a coping mechanism for a personal maturational crisis.

Clearly none of these theories completely explain the socio-cultural phenomena of eating disorders, they may assist with the identification of 'at risk' individuals.

Specific environmental and recreational factors whereby thinness is clearly linked with high achievement put certain individuals more at risk. For instance, models, gymnasts and dancers commonly manifest eating disorders, as do jockeys, wrestlers and distance runners. Male long-distance runners demonstrate behaviour patterns very akin to sufferers of anorexia nervosa with a continual preoccupation with food, emphasis on leanness, very high self-expectations and, like the other athletes mentioned, a marked denial of physical comfort in their quest for achievement.

The media, especially teenage and women's magazines, have been strongly criticised for promoting and reinforcing the thin-is-beautiful-and-successful concept. Photographs of glorified actresses and models who are artificially thin are published alongside articles on nutrition and recipes for the 'chocolate cake of the week', resulting in mixed messages about and confusing attitudes towards appearances and food.

The media should be applauded, however, for educating the public about a wide range of women's health issues, especially eating disorders. Anorexia nervosa and bulimia, like many other specific medical terms, are now household words. Most of the popular teenage magazines run excellent stories on sexuality, contraception, and nutrition. However, reducing the emphasis on thinness and pushing for a more holistic concept of health and beauty based on attributes other than weight would certainly contribute to the prevention of distorted body image and eating disorders in young women. Ultimately the prevention of eating disorders resides in our ability to change the socio-cultural conditions which promote anorexia and bulimia—namely the cultural value of thinness—and to promote self-esteem and good self-image.

As lifestyle and eating habits established in childhood usually persist throughout life, it is important that a rational attitude towards food, exercise and body image is established early on. A balanced diet without self-denial should be associated with a reasonable level of physical activity. The natural weight gain that accompanies puberty is important for, and compensated by, the growth spurt that occurs during adolescence. Children and adolescents should be given the psychological freedom to develop their own biologically normal weight. Obesity is usually a manifestation of fundamental lifestyle and psychological problems; however, the line between normal body weight and being overweight is becoming progressively blurred for the fast food generation of this century.

Finally, there is no denying that body image is an important component of self-esteem. It is possible to find a balance between body image, body weight and lifestyle. The point at which that balance occurs is different for different people, according to individual expectations and needs. Obviously a competitive gymnast is going to place more emphasis on his or her physique than others because body shape and appearance is integral to success in such an aesthetic sport. The rest of us should not feel guilty that we don't have the bodies of gymnasts or 'super-models'. On the other hand, body weight has a major impact on health. Women who are overweight are at greater risk of developing cardiovascular disease, breast cancer and endometrial cancer. Why this is so is considered in more detail in the chapters which deal with these diseases. Maintaining a body weight within the normal range is part of taking personal responsibility for our health. This is obviously easier for some than others, and certainly something often more easily said than done. However, being aware of eating patterns is a good start, and even small changes such as avoiding convenience food and cutting down on fat can make a big difference. Be positive and optimistic, think of your diet and exercise patterns from a health perspective and as a form of life insurance and consider the changes you can realistically make.

In summary, the aim of eating sensibly and being physically active is to achieve metabolic fitness and overall well-being, and to look good as a consequence of being fit and healthy.

3

DISORDERS OF MENSTRUATION

The menstrual cycle is an integral part of every woman's life and as a result has been the subject of many old wives' tales, myths and mystery. The menstrual cycle and menstruation are often treated in a negative manner, which is unfortunate because most women look forward to their reproductive years and lament their passing. Ovulation and menstruation affect women physically, psychologically and behaviourally and the experience is unique to each woman. Most women are aware of some fluctuations in their well-being during their natural cycle, but for the majority the changes experienced do not interfere with their lives. Some women, however, do experience menstrual disturbances, either psychological or physical, which impact significantly on their ability to function normally and relate to others.

It is impossible to consider difficulties with the menstrual cycle without initially reviewing when it usually begins and what is 'normal'. So here are some facts.

Young girls enter puberty at around ten years of age with an initial phase of accelerated growth and breast development known as breast budding. Shortly after, pubic hair appears, and by the age of twelve more than 50 per cent of young girls have underarm hair. By the age of twelve years and eight months 50 per cent have menstruated. However, the normal range of age for the onset starting periods is wide, being nine to seventeen years. The peak growth spurt occurs about a year before menstruation begins.

Ovulation is the release of a developed egg from the ovary into the fallopian tube. Most young women do not settle down to regular ovulatory cycles for two to three years after starting their periods. Even if the periods are occurring in a regular monthly pattern, many of the bleeds in the early years do not involve the production of a mature egg. Ovulation is a complex process and is influenced by numerous factors, both biological and psychological.

Hormones produced by the pituitary gland at the base of the brain are released into the blood stream and interact with the ovaries. The ovaries respond by the production of hormones known as oestrogens, progestogens and androgens, which in turn are released into the circulation and flow back to the central controls in the brain and the pituitary.

Ovulation only occurs when the brain, the pituitary gland and the ovaries are in balance. Physical or emotional stress can disrupt the balance, with some women being more susceptible than others. Examples of physical stress include regular strenuous exercise or weight loss.

Ovulation usually occurs on the fourteenth day of a 28 day cycle, although normal cycles vary in length from 21 to 35 days. Shorter or longer cycles are considered abnormal.

The first day of each cycle is designated as the first day of menstruation. Normal bleeding occurs for one to seven days. During this time a total of less than 80 mL (four tablespoons) of blood is lost. Losses greater than this are considered abnormal, as are the passing of clots during menstruation.

Bleeding between periods is also considered abnormal, although it is not uncommon for some women to have some very light transient blood loss, commonly known as 'spotting', just after ovulation. This appears to be related to the drop in oestrogen immediately following ovulation. Some women also experience spotting or break-through bleeding between periods when taking the oral contraceptive pill. This usually occurs because the oestrogen–progestogen balance in the pill being taken is not right for the affected woman. Changing to a different oral contraceptive which has a different oestrogen–

Brain control of the ovulatory cycle

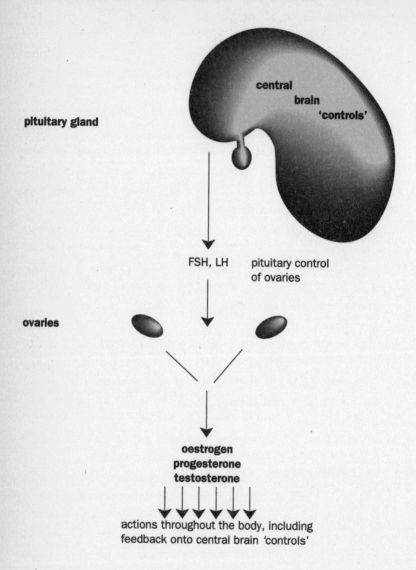

pituitary gland

central brain 'controls'

FSH, LH   pituitary control of ovaries

ovaries

oestrogen
progesterone
testosterone

actions throughout the body, including feedback onto central brain 'controls'

The pituitary gland, under the influence of important brain centres, releases the hormones FSH and LH. The amount of FSH and LH in the blood varies during the different stages of the menstrual cycle and it is the specific pattern of the release of these hormones that directs the ovaries through the monthly ovulatory cycle.

progestogen combination usually corrects the problem in most instances.

All abnormal uterine bleeding, whether prolonged or heavy menstruation or irregular mid-cycle bleeding, needs to be investigated. A Pap smear at least every two years is essential in all sexually active women, as well as a thorough pelvic examination. An ultrasound examination can be performed as an alternative way of preliminarily assessing the problem in women who have never been sexually active. The need for further investigations depends upon what is initially found. Iron deficiency is not uncommon in women with a history of heavy periods. A blood count (haemoglobin level) is not sufficient to rule out iron deficiency and specific iron studies including blood iron and a ferritin level (a measure of iron stores in the body) should be done.

The so-called 'disorders of menstruation' include severe symptoms of the normal menstrual cycle through to well-defined illness; however, frequently the boundaries between normal and abnormal are blurred. The most common problems associated with the menstrual cycle, apart from abnormal bleeding include:

- painful menstruation (dysmenorrhoea);
- premenstrual syndrome;
- menstrual migraine;
- menstrual epilepsy;
- irregular or absent menstruation (amenorrhoea).

AMENORRHOEA

There are many different causes of irregular or absent menstruation (amenorrhoea). Any teenager who has not started to menstruate by the age of sixteen years should consult a doctor and may need to have some investigations performed. It would be appropriate also to seek a medical opinion if more than three years has elapsed since breast development commenced without the onset of menstruation. Failure to menstruate can occur because of anatomical abnormalities, many of which are correctable, or can be due to a problem involving primarily the ovaries, the pituitary or the central brain control centre for ovulation, the hypothalamus. Alternatively, menstruation may commence normally but then the cycles can unexpectedly stop. There are several possible reasons why this may happen. Failure to menstruate completely is known as *primary amenorrhoea*, whereas cessation of established menstruation is called *secondary amenorrhoea*. The most common cause of primary amenorrhoea is a hereditary tendency towards late puberty, and such girls usually have a family history of either or both parents experiencing a late puberty. Initially no investigations or treatment is warranted in such circumstances (see also page 114).

Rather than give a broad overview of these causes of amenorrhoea, I focus specifically on the effects of exercise on the menstrual cycle later in this chapter. Many of the other issues concerning amenorrhoea are covered in Chapter 6. Let's now look at the other menstrual disorders.

PAINFUL MENSTRUATION

Premenstrual syndrome should not be confused, as is often the case, with premenstrual and menstrual pain, for which the correct medical term is *dysmenorrhoea*. (The direct Greek translation is 'difficult menstrual flow'.) Dysmenorrhoea (pronounced *dis–men–or–eah*) is severe, spasmodic, crampy, menstrual pain which is experienced deep in the lower back and lower abdomen pain, and which peaks just before and during the first 24 hours of heavy menstrual bleeding. Nausea, vomiting and diarrhoea often accompany the pain.

Surveys tell us that, overall, 60 per cent of adolescent girls suffer significant menstrual pain at some stage and fourteen per cent regularly miss school because of the severity of their menstrual symptoms. Painful menstruation is a feature of menstrual cycles in which ovulation occurs. As young girls frequently do not ovulate regularly, if at all, for the first two to three years following the start of their periods, painful periods are uncommon in the early teenage years. Significant menstrual pain is more of a problem in late adolescence and reportedly affects 72 per cent of seventeen-year-old females as opposed to less than 40 per cent of twelve-year-olds.

Interestingly, beyond late adolescence the frequency of reporting of severe menstrual pain decreases with age. This decline appears to be associated with young women becoming sexually active, irrespective of whether or not they are using the oral contraceptive pill.

WHAT CAUSES MENSTRUAL PAIN?

For many years it was believed that girls who suffered severe menstrual pain had primarily a psychological problem rather than a biological one. We are now aware that there is a biological chain of events which gives rise to the pain of menstruation, although some women do appear to suffer dysfunction that is out of proportion to the menstrual pain and other symptoms experienced. Psychological factors, such as stress or depression, will lower the pain threshold and cause decreased pain tolerance, and anxiety, stress and fear will also exacerbate the pain of menstruation. Similarly, other psychosocial problems, such as sexual anxiety or experiences of sexual abuse or other serious personal or family problems, can cause heightened anxiety about menstruation.

Cultural attitudes towards menstruation significantly affect the likelihood of experiencing menstrual pain. Many girls continue to enter puberty in trepidation of menstruation which has been considered a taboo, and experience their first bleeding with fear and shame, something to be hidden behind a locked door. Negative experiences such as stress and anxiety also may significantly increase the likelihood of a girl suffering painful menstruation.

Menstruation needs to be discussed positively and openly with young girls, they need to be encouraged to be proud of their bodies, their sexuality and reproductive capacity. Problematic menstrual pain is less common among females who have good health, high self-esteem and who are physically active.

The classic discomfort of menstruation has a biochemical basis. The lining of the uterus which is shed during menstruation, and the tissue fluid lost with it, contain chemicals called prostaglandins. These chemicals stimulate contraction of the uterus, resulting in pain. Women who experience very painful menstruation have been found to have higher than average prostaglandin levels. Alcohol and nicotine further increase menstrual cramps by their effects on the uterus. Period pain is sometimes classified as mild, moderate or severe to assist with treatment. Mild menstrual pain implies that pain only occurs during the first day of bleeding, there are minimal other symptoms and the individual can continue to function normally. Moderate dysmenorrhoea is used when pain lasts for two to three days with troublesome additional symptoms, for example nausea, vomiting, diarrhoea or headache, requiring time-out from usual activities. Severe menstrual pain, which affects five to ten per cent of menstruating women, significantly disrupts normal life.

Any girl or woman suffering moderate to severely painful menstruation should be medically assessed to make sure an underlying medical problem is not the cause for the pain. The extent of the medical examination necessary will vary according to the severity of the pain and whether or not the individual is sexually active. A Pap smear and samples for microbiology culture are essential for all sexually active women suffering significant menstrual pain to check for infections and changes in the cells of the cervix. Again, depending on whether the individual is sexually active, either a full pelvic examination or an abdominal ultrasound should be performed to exclude other abnormalities.

TREATMENT OF MENSTRUAL PAIN

Frequently, no specific medical intervention is necessary other than reassurance that no underlying disease exists. Evaluation of lifestyle factors is important and usually helpful, and consideration of the individual's attitudes or anxieties regarding menstruation is of value. It is vital that women attend a medical practitioner with whom they feel comfortable. *No* question is stupid. The more you ask, the more you will know and therefore the more you will be in control of your own body. It is impossible for your doctor to pre-empt all the questions in your mind, so help her or him by asking.

Anti-prostaglandin therapy

The mainstay of medical treatment is with a group of drugs called anti-inflammatory agents, which block the production of prostaglandins that cause the pain. To be effective, the tablets should be taken from the first sign of menstruation, which may be either pain or bleeding according to the individual. Starting treatment earlier does not appear to offer any advantage. The most commonly prescribed and effective agents are mefenamic acid, ibuprofen and naproxen. Treatment with these drugs results in pain relief in 60 to 95 per cent of women with an average reduction of 50 per cent.

Combined oral contraceptive pill (OCP)

Up to 50 per cent of women experience complete relief of menstrual pain with OCP use, and 30 to 40 per cent experience marked relief. The OCP blocks ovulation, thus the lining of the uterus stays fairly thin and the monthly production of the pain-inducing prostaglandins is reduced.

Combined treatment

Occasionally a combination of the OCP and an anti-prostaglandin is necessary to provide relief from menstrual pain in severely affected women.

Additional therapies

Rest, relaxation and massage or local heat to the lower back and pelvic area can be effective in relieving symptoms.

Black cohosh (see page 44) has been successfully prescribed for the management of menstrual pain. *Raspberry leaf tea*, an infusion prepared from the dried leaves of *Rubus idaeus L.*, has been advocated as a traditional therapy for menstrual pain and heavy bleeding. However there is limited evidence to support the effect of this remedy on the uterus and no clinical studies have been performed. Raspberry leaf tea appears to have several active constituents which result in opposing biological effects. It has been shown to contain chemicals which separately cause both smooth muscle stimulation and relaxation and it is not known which effect, if any, predominates on the uterus. Therefore the use of this therapy cannot be recommended on any sound scientific basis.

PREMENSTRUAL SYNDROME

The premenstrual syndrome was previously called *premenstrual tension* (PMT) or the *premenstrual tension syndrome* because of the tension and anxiety that feature as symptoms of this condition. Recognition of the diverse symptoms that women suffer premenstrually, however, has resulted in the currently used term *premenstrual syndrome* (PMS).

The validity of PMS as a genuine medical condition is controversial. The American Psychiatric Association published a set of precise diagnostic criteria for PMS in 1987 in an appendix to the *Diagnostic and Statistical Manual of Mental Disorders*, third edition. There is still, however, hot debate as to whether PMS is a biological entity or a social phenomenon. Clearly, cultural beliefs, social, environmental and educational factors are all important components governing the individual's understanding, expectation and experience of the menstrual cycle. It has been argued that focusing on the negative premenstrual changes increases the likelihood of women experiencing PMS. Some women report positive premenstrual changes with improved efficiency and creative energy during their premenstrual phase.

The legal implications of the diagnosis of PMS continues to evoke controversy. The diagnosis has been used either as a defence for women who have committed criminal acts or to implicate incompetence in cases involving civil matters.

Some research does indicate a link between mood and the hormonal changes of the menstrual cycle. Ovulation, which occurs in the middle of the cycle, is preceded by a surge in oestrogen. Many women report a heightened sense of well-being at this time. Ovulation is followed by an abrupt and brief fall in blood oestrogen levels and up to five per cent of women with PMS describe transient PMS-like symptoms of headache, depression or tension coinciding with the fall in oestrogen mid-cycle. After ovulation, progesterone production by the ovaries increases in order to prepare the uterus for a possible pregnancy. This interval between ovulation and the onset of menstruation, when progesterone is the 'dominant' hormone, is called the *luteal phase*. It is during this time many women experience the onset of premenstrual symptoms, which peak around the onset of menstruation. In contrast to popular belief, PMS symptoms do not immediately resolve when menstruation begins, even though oestrogen and progesterone levels have fallen. Some women are at their worst for the first 24 to 48 hours of menstruation and then experience resolution of their symptoms over the next few days. Others describe immediate relief of PMS within the first day of bleeding.

Some women experience no premenstrual symptoms, others minimal symptoms, while some are troubled for a day or two by mild to moderate problems. A minority of women (data from North America puts an estimate at three to eight per cent) suffer significant, disabling premenstrual symptoms, which can be classified as PMS, at some stage during their reproductive years.

The commonly described premenstrual symptoms include the following.

- *Weight gain*. Although a common complaint, there is no consistent data to support the occurrence of true weight gain premenstrually.
- *Abdominal bloating and constipation*. It has been proposed that the high levels of circulating blood progesterone in the luteal (premenstrual) phase affects the muscle layers of the bowel, causing bowel muscle relaxation and distension by fluid retention and gas. Hence some women experience abdominal bloating and their bowels may be more sluggish, resulting in constipation.
- *Fluid retention*. Many women have the sensation that they retain fluid premenstrually. 'Swollen', 'bloated' and 'distended' are commonly used adjectives. This has been difficult to document, but has been attributed to the increase in progesterone premenstrually. If fluid retention does occur, the extra water 'retained' is in the tissues not in the blood vessels. Diuretics (fluid tables) should not be used for premenstrual fluid. Diuretics remove excess water from the blood vessels and make users thirsty, resulting in increased water consumption and even further fluid retention.

The sensation of tissue swelling is a normal physiological symptom of a healthy reproductive cycle. Although some women are more sensitive to this than others, it is not a disorder of menstruation but a positive signal that ovulation has occurred and normal premenstrual progesterone is being produced.

- *Breast swelling and tenderness.* Again this is believed to be a progestogen effect.
- *Increased appetite compared with the other days of the cycle.* Many women experience specific food cravings, especially for sweet, calorie dense foods.
- *Reduced libido.* This may be a progestogen effect or due to a decline in oestrogen or testosterone. Premenstrually lessened libido is also caused or exacerbated by a negative body image experienced by some women during this phase and the feeling that they are less sexually attractive.
- *Headaches.* These range from mild through to full blown migraines (see the section on menstrual migraine).
- *Emotional instability.* Anxiety, nervous tension, irritability, depression, fatigue, reduced ability to concentrate, lowered self-esteem and a sense of being less able to cope are common complaints. The cause of these symptoms are at this stage not known.

True premenstrual syndrome can only be diagnosed when several of the above physical and psychological symptoms are experienced consistently in the premenstrual (luteal) days in the absence of any other medical condition or psychological illness. The recognised criteria for diagnosis of PMS therefore requires that:

- true PMS only occurs in women who ovulate;
- the symptoms must occur premenstrually, every month, with at least one symptom free week after each menstrual period;
- the symptoms are so severe that they interfere with the affected woman's work, domestic responsibilities and/or

her normal relationships; that is, the experience significantly affects and disrupts her normal life;

- an identifiable psychiatric disorder must be excluded.
Rarely a treatable psychiatric illness may initially appear
as PMS. For example, treatable depression may worsen
during the premenstrual days, but if correctly diagnosed
can be appropriately treated.

In order to clarify the link between the symptoms a
woman experiences and her menstrual cycle a menstrual diary
should be kept. Such a diary should include a list of troublesome symptoms, and daily over a period of at least three
months each of the symptoms can be considered and given
a numerical rating. For example, breast tenderness would be
rated as '0' when it did not occur, '1' for mild breast
tenderness through to '5' for 'It couldn't be worse!' By doing
such a chart both the affected woman and her physician can
objectively assess any symptom pattern and, equally importantly, assess the effect of any therapy used by the woman
during treatment. Charting symptoms over time is vital in
women who have had a hysterectomy, otherwise it is impossible to identify a cyclical pattern as there is no menstrual
loss to connect to the symptom.

The premenstrual syndrome is uncommon in adolescence.
It is a much greater problem for women in their thirties and
forties. Many women who have used the oral contraceptive
pill for a long time during their reproductive years and, who
decide to stop the pill for example in their forties, are taken
aback by their experience of PMS with resumption of ovulation. Such women also usually experience increased menstrual
loss after stopping the pill. This so-called increase is, in fact,
usually 'normal' menstrual loss but for the individual it is a
relative increase to the light periods previously experienced
on the combined pill.

In the years leading up to menopause, hormone fluctuations begin to occur, and commonly the menstrual cycle

becomes shorter. Many women experience premenstrual syndrome or menstrual migraines for the first time during these years.

Women suffering PMS frequently have underlying personality disorders or emotional tension. It is vital that all women with PMS carefully consider their life circumstances and try to identify, and if possible alleviate, any existing stressors. As for any disorder, just identifying and acknowledging relevant stress factor(s) is a major initial step. It is always much easier to deal with PMS if precipitating or exacerbating factors can be understood. However, PMS also affects many women who are otherwise healthy, well-adjusted individuals and it is wrong to label all PMS sufferers as environmentally stressed.

The cause of PMS is not known, despite extensive research addressing the psychological and hormonal aspects of this condition.

As outlined earlier, ovulation results from a complex series of interactions between the brain, the pituitary gland and the ovaries. Sex steroids chemically impact on normal brain function, particularly in the areas involved in mood (the limbic system), appetite and temperature regulation (the hypothalamus), as well as in centres of higher brain function important for memory and concentration. Some individuals are especially sensitive to the fluctuations that occur in the sex steroids oestrogen and progesterone during the menstrual cycle, as well as during or after pregnancy and menopause. Several studies have demonstrated that women who suffer severe PMS are more likely to have suffered post-natal depression and to experience problematic, menopausal, psychological symptoms in the future. Many women, in fact, relate the onset of their PMS to the menstrual cycles that followed their last pregnancy. A vast range of theories as to the cause of PMS have been proposed, but none have stood the tests of time or research. Theories have involved abnormal sensitivity to oestrogen, progesterone, adrenal hormones, pineal gland melatonin production, various pituitary gland hormones, as well as nutritional deficiencies of different vitamins and minerals.

It is possible for some women to continue to suffer PMS while taking the oral contraceptive pill. This is because either the low dose pill has not suppressed their natural cycle and they continue to ovulate, or because they are experiencing PMS-like side effects of the progesterone component of the combined oral contraceptive. This occurs more commonly with the 'triphasic' pills in which the dose of progestogen increases in three phases over the month, the highest dose of progestogen being in the premenstrual tablets. Women experiencing PMS on a triphasic pill usually benefit by changing to a constant dose (monophasic) oral contraceptive.

TREATMENT OF PMS

Although the cause of PMS is not known, various treatment strategies have been found by experience to alleviate some of the described symptoms. Treatment of PMS requires symptom documentation, pattern recognition and, most importantly, reassurance by the doctor and understanding by the affected woman that she is suffering genuine symptoms. Any specific treatment must be tailored to the individual in accordance with her needs, expectations and symptoms. The aim of any treatment is to improve well-being and the ability to function normally. Both women and doctors need to be aware that the management of this condition involves art more than science.

Lifestyle modification

Review of diet and exercise is important. Women should make sure they have a balanced diet low in fat and high in unrefined carbohydrate and fibre. Regular exercise will improve sleep patterns, enhance relaxation and reduce symptoms such as anxiety, tension and irritability. Many women benefit from counselling, stress reduction techniques and being formally taught how to be more assertive and in control of their lives.

The combined oral contraceptive pill

The OCP suppresses natural ovulation and for many women results in relief of symptoms. A continuous, unvarying dose (monophasic) OCP is preferable to one of the triphasic pills.

Other hormonal manipulation

A potent, synthetic hormone called Duphaston is sometimes effective in women with severe symptoms. Alternatively, the ovaries can be totally switched off by the administration of a type of drug called a GnRH-agonist and then low dose oestrogen replacement given. However, these are radical temporary treatments that should not be used routinely.

Fluoxetine (Prozac)

A drug used to treat depression has been found to be extremely effective as a treatment for women suffering severe, psychological PMS symptoms. The mechanism by which Prozac lessens the psychological symptoms of PMS appears to be different from its anti-depressant action. When taken as an anti-depressant, the beneficial effects of Prozac are not experienced for several weeks. In contrast, when used to alleviate PMS the effects of Prozac are immediate; that is, they are experienced in the first month of use, and the benefits are achieved with a much lower dose than that needed for the anti-depressant action.

Prozac can be taken continuously; however, it appears to be equally effective when taken each month from day fourteen of the cycle (mid-cycle) until menstruation. Taken in this way and in a low dose (20 mg) the likelihood of developing dependence on Prozac is remote.

Natural therapies

Various natural therapies are prescribed to alleviate the symptoms of PMS. Therapies shown to be no better than a placebo (a sugar tablet) in controlled scientific studies include vitamin B6 and evening primrose oil.

Evening primrose oil (EPO) is refined from the small seed of the native American wildflower *Oenothera Biennis L.* It has become highly regarded as an effective therapy for breast tenderness and other PMS symptoms. However, formal medical research has shown EPO to be no more effective than placebo tablets in the treatment of this symptom. In view of this, and its considerable expense, its use cannot be endorsed (see also page 92).

Borage seed oil, refined from the seed of *Borago Officinalis L.,* contains similar oils to evening primrose oil. It also contains toxic alkaloids which can cause liver damage and therefore its use cannot be recommended.

Extracts of the fruit of the *chaste berry tree*, *Vitex agnus-castus L.,* is sometimes prescribed for PMS and menopausal symptoms. However efficacy has not been established and awaits further evaluation. Sensitive individuals can develop an itchy rash from the extract.

Black cohosh is also known as black snakeroot or cimicifuga from the plant *Cimicifuga racemosa L.* Extracts of black cohosh have been shown to have oestrogen-like activity with use resulting in a reduction in menopausal hot flushes. It may be effective in the treatment of PMS. It is usually taken in the form of a 40 to 60 per cent alcoholic extract. It may cause stomach upsets, but no major complications have been reported with its use. Because no long-term studies on the safety of black cohosh have been performed, however, its use should be limited to six months or less.

MENSTRUAL MIGRAINE

Headache, one of the most commonly suffered medical symptoms, is reported disproportionately more by women than by men. Women not only experience more headaches but also suffer more severe pain. A menstrual link should be considered for every woman who has frequent headaches. A definitive pattern can only be determined by keeping a calendar of the headaches and associated symptoms and evaluating their occurrence in relationship to menstruation. The connection must be clearly documented in order initially to make a diagnosis of premenstrual or menstrual headache and subsequently to evaluate the efficacy of any therapy.

Menstrual migraine can be defined as cyclical, severe headache which begins at the onset of or during menstruation. Alternatively, cyclical headaches may occur premenstrually and are classified as part of the premenstrual syndrome. Sixty per cent of female migraine sufferers report an association with their migraines and menstruation and fourteen per cent of women with migraine only experience headaches during menstruation.

Premenstrual headache differs from menstrual migraine in that it appears to be caused by prostaglandins, the levels of which rise before and at the start of menstruation (see the section on premenstrual syndrome). Prostaglandins have direct effects on the blood-vessels with different types of prostaglandins causing blood-vessel constriction and dilation, as well as increasing the sensitivity of blood-vessel walls to pain.

Menstrual migraine is believed to result from the precipitous decline in hormone levels at the onset of menstruation. Increased circulating prostaglandin levels probably also play a role in menstrual migraine; however, the majority of women suffering menstrual migraine experience this as a specific problem and do not complain of PMS.

Usually the headaches are classic migraine with frequent visual disturbances, light sensitivity, nausea and debilitating pain, although there is considerable variation between individuals.

TREATMENT OF MENSTRUAL MIGRAINE

Diagnosis depends on clearly documenting a relationship between headaches and menstruation over a period of at least three months. As for all cases of recurrent migraine, lifestyle and dietary factors that may impact on the severity of headaches need to be reviewed. Things to avoid include alcohol, cigarettes, caffeine and excessive fatigue. By the time the diagnosis of menstrual migraine is made, most women have tried all these standard lifestyle modification strategies.

The most effective medications for a menstrual migraine that has already developed are anti-prostaglandin agents, also known as nonsteroidal anti-inflammatory drugs (NSAIDs), such as naproxen sodium, mefenamic acid or ibuprofen. A reduction in the severity and duration of headache with use of any of these medications, as well as alleviation of the associated symptoms of nausea, vomiting and visual disturbances, has been established.

Obviously, preventing attacks is preferabe to treating an established headache. Effective options include the following.

- Use of a 'natural', oral oestrogen or an oestrogen skin patch commencing just prior to menstruation and continuing for seven days. The dose should be tapered at the end of the treatment period to prevent rebound headache.
- Continuous low dose, combined oral contraceptive pill use; that is, not stopping for one week, or taking the sugar tablets, but continuing straight on to the next pack of active pills. Some women develop 'break-through bleeding' with this therapy or are concerned that by not

having a period they can't be sure they are not pregnant. An effective alternative is use of the oral contraceptive pill with additional natural oestrogen therapy during the one-week break. An example of this would be three weeks of the OCP and then 0.625–1.25 mg of Premarin (oestrogen) for one week before the next three weeks of the OCP. Again, a woman needs to check with her treating doctor what is right for her.

MENSTRUAL EPILEPSY

The best definition of menstrual epilepsy is seizures occurring predominantly at, or exacerbated by, menstruation. A relationship between the menstrual cycle and seizure occurrence has been noted in up to 70 per cent of women who continue to suffer epileptic seizures. There appear to be two peaks of enhanced epileptic risk: at mid-cycle and from the onset of menstruation.

Research into hormones and the occurrence of epilepsy indicates possible roles for both oestrogens and progestogens. It has been suggested that progesterone may have an anti-epileptic effect, that menstrual epilepsy is precipitated by the sudden fall in progesterone levels just prior to menstruation and that treatment with synthetic progestogens, (medroxyprogesterone acetate or norethisterone) may reduce epileptic attacks in women with menstrual epilepsy. Oestrogens, on the other hand, may enhance epileptic activity in the brain. However, none of this has been conclusively demonstrated. It could be equally argued that mid-cycle and menstrual epilepsy is precipitated by the fall in oestrogen levels observed at both of these phases of the cycle.

Premenstrual water retention has also been proposed as a cause for menstrual epilepsy. As this appears to be a predominantly progestogen effect it is in conflict with the concept that progestogens are anti-epileptic.

A particular diuretic, acetazolamide (Diamox), may be effective in preventing menstrual epilepsy when taken for ten days before the expected start of menstruation, and continued until bleeding ends. The usually recommended dose is 250 to 500 mg per day. No formal study has been conducted to establish the value of this line of management. The main side effects of Diamox include drowsiness and tingling in the extremities.

A more conservative approach for women who experience cyclic menstrual epilepsy is increasing the dose of the prescribed daily anti-epileptic medication for the week before menstruation and returning to the usual dose when bleeding ceases. Clearly, the dose variation must be managed by the treating physician.

Hormonal manipulation is only indicated in a small number of women and requires the input of either a hormone specialist (endocrinologist) or a gynaecologist with an interest in this condition.

EXERCISE AND MENSTRUATION

Reproductive problems are common among elite female athletes, especially when their rigorous training program is compounded by weight loss. The disorders such women develop are complete failure to menstruate, which means they are not ovulating, or more subtle cycle defects in which cycles appear to be regular or only slightly abnormal but, in fact, the hormonal levels are subnormal and ovulation doesn't occur. Young athletes frequently have delayed puberty or, of more concern, may even fail to menstruate at all by their late teenage years because of the impact of their training on their reproductive cycle (see page 49). The long-term consequences of this type of reproductive dysfunction in elite athletes result from their being deficient in the important sex hormones oestrogen and progesterone.

Long-term failure to ovulate, and therefore chronically low oestrogen and progesterone levels, may lead to bone loss, fractures, especially stress fractures, and ultimately osteoporosis. Whereas moderate exercise results in an increase in bone density in most women, the combination of excessive exercise and low oestrogen leads to bone loss. A good example is a 24-year-old female triathlete who stopped menstruating because of her increased exercise, but was found to have normal bone density for her age. After a further twelve months of continued intensive training, two to three hours each day, a repeat bone density study demonstrated she had lost five per cent of her bone mass over that time frame. Bone loss does not occur in elite athletes who continue to menstruate regularly and therefore have normal oestrogen levels. Low body weight and exercise do not cause the bone loss—the problem resides in the lack of oestrogen. In fact, the intensive weight bearing activity of gymnastics is a powerful stimulus for bone formation, and young female gymnasts with regular menstrual cycles have stronger bones than their non-athletic counterparts.

Infertility can be another problem related to intensive exercise programs and, contrary to the general belief that exercise always lowers cholesterol, some of these women, in fact, have abnormal blood fat levels as a result of their oestrogen deficiency. The long-term significance of this has not been studied. The prevalence of this problem of exercise interfering with normal menstrual cycles in women has increased over the last few decades with the growing involvement of women in endurance sports. In 1970 only one woman ran the New York City Marathon and she did not finish the race. In 1990 5249 women entered the same marathon and 4500 finished. Female long-distance runners often report running 70 or more miles per week as their regular training program. In some, but certainly not all, studies menstrual irregularities have been observed to increase with the greater the distance run.

Runners are certainly not the only women affected. Women engaged in other sports in which low body weight is an advantage for both aesthetics and enhanced performance, such as ballet dancers, gymnasts and figure skaters, are also at high risk of menstrual abnormalities. Dancers and gymnasts spend many hours every week in rigorous training programs and usually have below normal body weight. Disorders of menstruation usually affect two to five per cent of the general female population, but have been observed in up to 51 per cent of females involved in one of these disciplines. Various factors including both the physical and mental stress of the training, particularly at a competitive level, may precipitate the menstrual disturbances. The common mechanism which ultimately causes disturbed cycles is suppression of the brain signals to the pituitary gland which then fails to stimulate the ovaries (see page 29). Because there is nothing fundamentally wrong with the ovaries—that is, they are just 'switched off' by failure of the correct signals to get through—these menstrual abnormalities are usually reversible.

The specific factors which combine to suppress the brain signals include stress, diet and weight loss.

Ballet dancers and gymnasts not only have low body weight but also commonly exhibit inappropriate attitudes toward food and eating disorders. The pressure to be thin for an appearance which is seen as synonymous with success is clearly manifested in these disciplines which involve girls from a young age. Many of them have eating patterns akin to sufferers of anorexia nervosa. A high intake of fibre is also common among ballet dancers who fail to have periods. The high fibre diet is filling and low fat, but also is associated with low oestrogen levels, as the fibre binds bile oestrogens which are then excreted instead of being reabsorbed. Similarly, dietary calcium becomes bound up in the dietary fibre and excreted rather than absorbed. Therefore these girls are at the added risk of bone loss because of the interaction between their oestrogen deficiency and poor dietary calcium absorption. Female gymnasts who ultimately achieve success in their discipline commence extended hours of intense training at a young age. Whether it is ethical for young girls to be subjected to such psychological and mental stress during their prepubertal years is questionable. It certainly seems incongruous that many of the elite female gymnasts who delight the world with their amazing, aesthetically pleasing performances have subjected themselves to disruption of their own natural growth and pubertal development to achieve this end.

Body weight is another important variable in the equation. Athletes who are ten to twelve per cent below ideal body weight are at the greatest risk of ovulatory disturbances. Fat stores are gender specific, with women tending to carry fat around the hips and thighs whereas men collect it more centrally around the abdomen. Depletion of hip and thigh fat may signal to the brain that there are inadequate fat reserves for normal reproductive function, i.e., pregnancy and lactation, and the brain then switches off the ovulatory signals. Retention of normal female fat distribution may be more important than maintaining 'normal' total body fat. It has been proposed that women need to have at least 22 per cent of their body mass as fat to have regular cycles, although, female athletes with less than seventeen per cent body fat often have regular cycles.

I believe the fundamental factor determining whether an individual elite female athlete will experience ovulatory dysfunction is the degree to which she is physically and mentally stressed and the sensitivity of her central brain receptors to that stress. Young women with immature message pathways between the brain, the pituitary gland and the ovaries appear to be more susceptible to the stresses arising from extreme training. Women who have experienced a pregnancy, and therefore have well-established reproductive message pathways, have been found to be less likely to develop menstrual problems with endurance training. This again brings into question the ethics of prepubertal girls participating in ongoing, intense athletic training programs.

Interestingly, men who engage in long-distance running have also been found to have various hormonal abnormalities. Some, but not all, studies have found that male marathon runners have depressed testosterone (male hormone) levels. One study in particular of men who had been regularly running between 125 to 200 km per week for at least five years found that their patterns of pituitary hormone release were strikingly similar to those observed in female athletes with menstrual problems. (The pituitary hormones stimulate the testes to produce testosterone and make sperm in men akin to the pituitary stimulating the ovaries to produce oestrogen and ovulation in women). Another study of male runners found that elite male, long-distance runners had significantly lower bone density of the spine, thigh bones and total body than non-runners. The further a man ran per week, the lower his bone density. Men who ran more than 100 km had on average nineteen per cent less bone mineral content (bone strength) than non-runners! Thus the impact of elite athletic training on reproductive hormones and the skeleton is not limited to women. This is one aspect that has been less studied in men than in women and the mechanism by which intensive exercise training affects men is not at present clear.

Until recently, competitive female swimmers were not believed to be subject to menstrual disturbances as a result of their training. Swimming is a non-weight bearing exercise for which thinness is not an advantage or a feature. It is considered a weight-supported activity in which increased muscle mass correlates with performance capacity. Elite swimmers generally weigh more and have a greater percentage of their body mass as fat than runners. However, swimmers also usually start dedicated training at a very young age and are subject to intense physical and mental stress well before their reproductive system has had a chance to mature. Competitive swimmers frequently experience delayed puberty when compared with normal girls and 82 per cent of adolescent swimmers have menstrual abnormalities in contrast to 40 per cent of aged-matched young women.

The mechanism causing the menstrual problems in swimmers differs from that of runners in that the swimmers have normal oestrogen levels and normal to high pituitary hormone levels. The dysfunction appears to be in the ovarian and adrenal production of hormones, so that excessive amounts of specific hormones called *pre-androgens*, made by the adrenal glands, are produced and these hormones appear to interfere with the processes required for normal ovulation.

It may well be that the women who perform best at different sports do so because of their genetic predisposition for the specific activities involved. They also may have in their genetic make-up a susceptibility to develop the different types of ovulatory disturbance inherent in the various sports. For example, swimmers require a different body build to runners. The genetic make-up which results in the body build of successful female swimmers may also be linked to the genes that make swimmers more likely to develop dysfunction of the ovaries. So the problem may be one of having a fundamental genetic predisposition to abnormalities of ovarian function which is unmasked by the process of swimming training.

Similarly, individuals with a particular body shape, not too tall and lean, are more likely to be good distance runners. This genetically predetermined physique may be linked to a sensitivity to menstrual disturbances.

Finally, all elite athletes tend to have certain psychological characteristics which include the ability to focus, determination, application and toleration of the physical pain associated with endurance training. Individuals with these attributes may be more susceptible to interruption of the brain signals to the pituitary, and hence central nervous system disruption of ovulation.

DEALING WITH MENSTRUAL DISTURBANCES

Long-term oestrogen deficiency is an abnormal state for young women and should be considered seriously. Nearly all elite athletes will resume normal ovulatory function if they exercise less and eat more, but understandably few are willing to do so, especially when approaching their peak. The simplest medical option is hormone replacement. The controversy that surrounds the use of hormone replacement therapy (HRT) after menopause is not relevant in this setting. It is normal for young women to have oestrogen circulating in their bodies, and lack of oestrogen during the reproductive years is a hormone deficiency with significant consequences, the most important being loss of bone.

Providing oestrogen replacement for a young woman whose body has stopped producing a sufficient amount for good health is comparable to giving thyroid hormone replacement to a person with thyroid gland failure and insulin to a diabetic. The debate surrounding the use of HRT in later years concerns whether or not it is appropriate to extend the time which a woman's body is naturally exposed to oestrogen, that is after the natural end to the reproductive years, and the risks and benefits of such therapy. This is an entirely different issue.

Hormone replacement can be in the form of either natural hormone replacement therapy or the oral contraceptive pill. If contraception is required, clearly the OCP is the obvious choice. An accepted doctrine is that young women need more oestrogen and progestogen for adequate replacement than post-menopausal women. Some doctors advocate that to achieve this it is necessary to use the OCP. I believe, however, that if contraception is not an issue, natural oestrogens are the preferred option with cyclical progestogen, ideally *medroxyprogesterone acetate* (Provera) or *micronized progesterone*, given in adequate doses (see Chapter 6).

Some women are reluctant to take any hormone therapy. This is understandable for several reasons. They don't want their body shape to change as this may be detrimental to their perceived success. They are often apprehensive about induction of menstruation. Teenagers with a prepubescent physique who are performing as ballet dancers and gymnasts need to discuss their femininity and body image and explore their attitude to their bodies, as well as consider the health consequences of their oestrogen deficiency state. Attitudes towards eating and food and peer group pressures complicate their treatment. Fear that hormones will make them want to eat more, and that hormones make people fat is common. In the aesthetic sports in particular body image is inseparable from self-esteem and the ability to achieve.

Any girl in this category who has menstrual difficulties must find a doctor who not only has a good understanding of the medical issues involved but who also has a compassionate, empathetic attitude so that the affected girl feels she can honestly discuss the issues important to her, and what she wants as a result of any treatment.

When hormone replacement is contraindicated other treatment regimes can be used to prevent bone loss, for example the use of bisphosphonates which prevent bone reabsorption. This is not optimal therapy, however, and should be limited to a select group of young women. Whether swimmers ultimately encounter the same problems as runners in terms of bone loss is not known, but it is unlikely because they have adequate circulating oestrogen. All female elite swimmers who experience menstrual irregularities need to be formally medically assessed and investigated with any required treatment suggested by the findings.

The determination, perseverance and skill required by people, particularly young women, to achieve elite athletic status requires community respect and support. These young women need not only encouragement but also understanding of their attitudes towards their endeavours and medical backup to optimise immediate and long-term good health.

4
'HIRSUTISM'—THE BODY HAIR DILEMMA

As we have already discussed, body image is an important component of self-esteem. Anxiety about appearances, which basically translates into body image, is the main factor governing women's attitudes towards their body hair. Many women are troubled by what they feel to be excess or an undesirable distribution or amounts of body hair. Individual expectations and acceptance of what constitutes 'normal' in terms of female body hair varies considerably. In general, women in Westernised countries have become attuned to the concept that having minimal facial and body hair is more attractive, and utilise a range of cosmetic techniques to cover up or remove unwanted hair.

Normal body hair growth is determined genetically and differs both within and between different racial groups. The uncertainty and anxiety about normality in terms of body hair may not be so great in genetically homogenous populations, for example among Greek women living in Greece. However in countries with mixed populations such as Australia, where immigrants have come from all parts of the world, differences between ethnic groups in terms of the acceptability of female body hair are amplified. A degree of hairiness which may be acceptable in the country of someone's genetic origin may not be acceptable to either that individual or the general community in a different country. Furthermore, body hair is less of a social issue in environments where women are more extensively covered by clothing according to religion or tradition or necessity, such as in a cold climate. In an environment where standards of dress for women are more liberal, the climate is warm and participation in sports, particularly swimming, is the norm, women are more likely to be anxious about hair growing on their upper thighs, abdomen or back. So the problem of body hair must be considered not only in terms of what is biologically normal or abnormal but also according to various social environments.

In our society, so oriented towards optimising physical appearances, the psychological and social impact of undesirable hairiness in a girl or woman cannot be underestimated or trivialised. For too many women it is a great source of anxiety, leading to low self-esteem and restrictions in lifestyle. Furthermore, individual expectations and acceptance of what is 'normal' or tolerable must be taken into account. Excessive body hair is infrequently a manifestation of an underlying hormonal disorder, which if treated may result in less hair growth. Therefore, it is more than reasonable for women who feel they have a problem with body hair to seek medical assessment. Understanding what is normal versus abnormal for female body hair, as opposed to what is cosmetically desirable, can be difficult as well as confusing.

In Australia, approximately nine per cent of women over the age of fourteen feel they have excessive body hair and, of these, one-quarter are considerably troubled by their problem. For most women unwanted facial hair generates the greatest anxiety.

Women usually develop their awareness of body hair on entering puberty as their body image begins to develop. A typical story is that of a young girl who was extremely athletic and enjoyed being the Sports Captain for her primary school. Around the time she entered puberty her family moved to a different city and she commenced secondary education at a co-educational school. Her anxiety about her increasing body hair was heightened by the presence of boys at the school. She recalls deliberately losing running races in order not to be selected for the school team as she was so self-conscious in her scanty sports uniform. She gave up swimming and on purpose continued to underachieve in sport to avoid embarrassment. She now is intensely aware of the impact her anxiety regarding her body hair had on her involvement in sport at school and her socialisation. She sends her daughters to an all-girl's school for several reasons, an important one being to minimise their self-consciousness of their impending pubertal development. She is hopeful they will be able to participate in the activities of their choice unencumbered by anxiety about their physical appearance.

This is only one of many stories I have heard over the years. Every week I encounter young women who will not wear shorts or go to the beach with friends because they are embarrassed by their 'hairy' thighs and arms. It is not just that they don't feel beautiful, they are often worried that people will think they have hormonal problems and that their appearance is too masculine. So this is not about body hair in a feminist context, or women in general having to conform to society's expectation that women should have shaved underarms and legs. The affected girls and women just want to be like their 'normal' female counterparts. Instead, they have male pattern facial hair growth or heavy abdominal hair growth or pubic hair extending over their upper thighs. Their genetically determined 'normal' body hair is different from their friends'. They feel they must hide their difference and thus their problem of body hair becomes socially disabling.

NORMAL BODY HAIR

The number of hair follicles we have is genetically programmed and fixed before birth. Hair follicles are found all over the body except for the palms, lips and soles of the feet. Most body hair is fine and unpigmented. Body hair growth is governed by the action of sex hormones on the hair follicles. Not only are the absolute levels of sex hormones in the blood important but also the sensitivity of the hair follicles to the hormones. Thus two women with the same blood hormone levels will have different body hair growth patterns according to the number of hair follicles over their bodies and the sensitivity of their hair follicles to the growth stimulating effects of the hormones.

The main hormones stimulating hair growth are called *androgens*. Androgens are commonly called 'male hormones', but this is somewhat misleading as androgens are normally produced by both the adrenal glands and ovaries in women and have important actions in normal healthy women.

The adrenal glands sit above the kidneys and, as well as producing androgens, produce the important 'stress' hormones cortisol and adrenaline. The most well-known androgen is *testosterone*. Testosterone is converted to oestrogen in the ovaries and body fat. Women cannot make oestrogen unless they can first make testosterone or adrenal androgens.

The other weaker androgens which are made by both the adrenal glands as well as the ovaries circulate in the blood stream. They are converted to both testosterone and oestrogen in other parts of the body and are major sources of blood testosterone in women of all ages, and oestrogen in postmenopausal women. The skin and hair follicles convert these androgens to testosterone, therefore high levels of these weak androgens, usually due to adrenal gland overactivity, can cause acne and excessive hair growth.

Hair follicles in certain parts of the body are more sensitive to the influence of androgens and are called the hormone or androgen sensitive areas of the body. These areas include the upper lip, sides of the face, chin, central chest and around the nipples, lower abdomen, back, upper arms, pubic region and inner thighs. In contrast, the arms and lower legs are less sensitive to the effects of hormones. Androgens not only stimulate hair growth in the hormone sensitive areas by increasing the speed of hair growth but also increase the pigmentation (darkening) of hair and the thickness of the hairs. Thus androgens convert fine, unpigmented hair into coarser, dark, more rapidly growing hair.

The medical term *hirsutism* is used to describe the condition of excessive, thick, dark hair growth in women in the androgen sensitive regions of the body in a pattern not considered normal for a woman.

Again the issue is not straightforward. Two girls may have the same pattern and extent of body hair. One may have normal blood hormone levels and normal body hair growth for her biological make-up. The second girl may have abnormally high androgen levels with abnormal body hair growth that is not in keeping with her natural biological constitution. This is because an equivalent amount of body hair may be a sign of a disease process in some women yet be genetically normal for others. The problem therefore is, where does normal end and abnormal begin?

Puberty begins with the development of underarm and pubic hair. This sexual hair starts to appear when the adrenal glands 'switch on' and produce increasing amounts of androgens at the onset of puberty. We do not know what triggers this initial phase of maturation. By the end of puberty there is considerable variation in the amount of body hair between individuals. As women age, their overall amount of coarse body hair tends to gradually increase, again with a wide range of individual variation.

WHEN IS HAIR GROWTH EXCESSIVE?

Any woman who feels she has excessive facial or body hair, that is feels she has more than a minor cosmetic nuisance, should seek medical assessment and advice. An underlying hormonal disorder is more likely in women who have irregular periods or acne. Often women have a family history of excessive body hair which clearly indicates a genetic component, although this does not help distinguish whether or not there is an underlying problem. A sudden increase in body hair, especially if associated with acne, is a cause for concern and indicates the need for investigations to be carried out. Other specific signs of abnormal hormone levels include deepening of the voice, loss of scalp hair in a pattern similar to balding in men and an increase in libido. Hirsutism may also be linked to obesity and diabetes in some women (see the section on polycystic ovarian syndrome on page 62).

It is obviously difficult to assess the severity of a woman's hirsutism. Doctors use a scoring system devised many years ago by the researchers Ferriman and Gallway. The system is quite simple. The body is considered as nine separate regions and the extent of hair in each region is given a value ranging from zero for no hair to four for complete coverage of hair equivalent to male pattern growth. A score above eight indicates hair growth in excess of that expected for a woman, whereas the problem is described as severe when a woman is given a score greater than nineteen. Although this scoring system has major limitations it is about the only method of clinical assessment available to doctors and provides at least a yard-stick for judging any response to medical treatment.

WHAT CAUSES INCREASED HAIR GROWTH?

Most women with the problem of hirsutism do not have a specific hormonal abnormality and are said to have *spontaneous* hirsutism. Blood tests may reveal slightly increased levels of androgen hormones, but more commonly blood tests are normal. Blood hormone levels tell us nothing about hormone production or the sensitivity of the skin and hair follicles to the hormones. However, research indicates that many women with hirsutism and normal blood hormone levels in fact have increased androgen turnover and/or enhanced sensitivity to normal levels of circulating hormones.

Polycystic ovarian syndrome (PCO) is the most commonly identified condition causing excessive hair growth in women. PCO is common and classically develops after puberty when girls experience irregular, infrequent periods. The progressive increase in body hair is usually associated with weight gain. Acne is also a common feature. The name of this condition is misleading. The ovaries are not actually full of cysts but contain excessive numbers of *follicles*, which are best described as 'mini cysts' which develop as a result of failed ovulation. In simple terms, certain cells in the ovaries of women with PCO overproduce androgens especially testosterone. These high levels of androgens, in the ovaries interfere with the development of a normal egg and, instead of normal ovulation proceeding, the nest of cells or the follicle containing the developing egg turns into a mini cyst. These mini cysts are clearly identified by an ultrasound examination. It is essential that the diagnosis of PCO is made by someone experienced in ultrasound of the ovaries. PCO can easily be confused with multicystic ovaries, which is a biological variation of normal and does not appear to be related to hormonal imbalance. Whereas a normal ovary contains up to three small follicles the ovaries of women with PCO contain ten or more follicles. This condition appears to affect up to twenty per cent of women with varying degrees of severity. Women who have both PCO and a problem with weight are more likely to have higher androgen levels, excessive body hair and problems with infertility. Women with PCO and obesity usually have high blood insulin levels and are at significant risk of developing diabetes.

The best treatment for PCO is weight control. Overweight girls with PCO who have absent or irregular periods often find their menstrual cycles become regular, their hormone levels normalise and their body hair diminishes if they lose weight. Girls with normal body weight and PCO may be less likely to run into major problems of infertility if they can keep their weight down. The problem of excessive body hair or acne can be treated with specific anti-androgen medication (see below). Such treatment deals only with the hair growth and acne, it does not treat the underlying ovarian problem. We don't know the specific cause of PCO other than it appears to be an inherited condition.

The next most common medical condition causing excessive body hair growth is *congenital adrenal hyperplasia* (CAH). This is an inherited condition usually diagnosed in childhood. More subtle forms may not appear, however, until after puberty as increased body hair in women. When this occurs it is called *late-onset CAH*. This condition is more common in certain ethnic groups and can be diagnosed with specific blood tests.

Rarely excessive body hair growth is caused by overproduction of one of the *pituitary hormones*, such as growth hormone, prolactin, or the adrenal stimulating hormone, ACTH. Usually other identifying abnormal symptoms and signs are present and specialised blood tests lead to the correct diagnosis.

Tumours or cancer growths which produce abnormal quantities of androgens are fortunately extremely rare. They are usually associated with a sudden and significant increase in hair growth and other signs of masculinisation.

Some *medications* can cause an increase in body hair, the most commonly prescribed one being phenytoin (Dilantin) which is used in the treatment of epilepsy.

WHAT TESTS SHOULD BE DONE?

As most women with hirsutism do *not* have a major underlying disease causing their problem, few blood tests are necessary.

- Women with mild to moderate excessive hair growth which has developed gradually and who have regular periods do not need any investigations.
- Women with more extensive hair growth (severe hirsutism) and regular periods should have their blood androgen levels measured.
- Women with increased hair growth and irregular periods need to have more extensive blood hormone tests done.

Most women with moderate to severe hirsutism should have their ovaries viewed by ultrasound, especially if they have irregular menstrual cycles. Ideally, a vaginal ultrasound should be performed as the ovaries are seen more clearly when the study is done in this manner. A vaginal ultrasound study is neither uncomfortable or overly invasive when performed by someone trained in this technique. The diagnosis of PCO is frequently missed when an abdominal ultrasound is done, and then picked up when a vaginal ultrasound is performed later.

The need for other specialised tests is determined by the results of the initial investigations.

MANAGEMENT OF HIRSUTISM

There is no instant or permanent cure for hirsutism. Once possible underlying diseases have been ruled out, management options can be considered. The aim of any therapy for hirsutism is for the affected woman to achieve a physical appearance and body image that she finds personally acceptable. This may be done by either cosmetic measures or the use of medications or sometimes a combination of both.

It is vital to understand that management is long term and every woman must choose a plan which she feels she can maintain over an extended period.

Of the available cosmetic measures, plucking, waxing and the use of hair removal (depilatory) creams are the simplest and most reliable and accessible options. Shaving is believed by many to enhance hair growth but this is not the case. After shaving the blunted cut edge of the shaved hairs re-emerge giving the impression that the hair has thickened up. Most women understandably prefer not to shave when their problem is of excessive facial hair, as this practice tends to reinforce an undesirable masculinised image.

Although expensive and time consuming, electrolysis can be extremely successful when performed by an experienced professional. However, multiple treatments over many months are required to achieve permenant hair removal. The efficiency of electrolysis may be increased when performed in combination with prescribed medical treatment.

Obese women suffering from hirsutism, particularly those with polycystic ovaries, often achieve a dramatic reversal of their problem with weight reduction. Loss of weight may result in hormonal levels returning to normal, lessened body hair growth and frequently the return of regular menstruation.

DRUG TREATMENT OF HIRSUTISM

The drugs used to treat excessive hair growth act by either blocking the action of androgens on hair growth or by reducing the production of androgens by the ovaries and adrenals.

The average length of a cycle of growth for a single hair follicle of the face, body and extremities ranges from two to three months. A full cycle must be complete before changes in the growth characteristics of a hair can be observed, that is either thickening and darkening with androgen excess or thinning and lightening with anti-androgen therapy. This means that whatever therapy is used, it takes at least six months before any positive changes can be seen. During the early treatment phase, the hair follicles may pass through one or more growth cycles and as they do so the growth blocking effect of the therapy gradually becomes apparent. The full effect of treatment cannot be judged until at least twelve months of treatment has been completed. Therefore, women considering drug therapy for hirsutism, need to be prepared to commit themselves to at least one year of treatment. Furthermore, drugs taken to decrease hair growth are only effective as long as the drug is taken, after which the original growth pattern of the hair follicle re-emerges.

The combined oral contraceptive pill reduces hormone production by the ovaries and is quite effective in reducing hair growth in many women. The new oral contraceptive pills are probably the most effective.

The other prescribed medications are called anti-androgens since, in various ways, they block androgen stimulation of body hair growth. Reduction of scalp hair growth is not a side effect; in fact, anti-androgens are prescribed to decrease scalp hair loss caused by abnormal hormonal actions. Approximately 80 per cent of women with hirsutism will experience an improvement with drug therapy. In North America the most frequently prescribed anti-androgen is *spironolactone* (Aldactone). Spironolactone is taken as a tablet every day. Women with irregular menstrual cycles often begin to ovulate regularly when taking this drug. In contrast, women who already have regular periods may develop irregular periods with this treatment.

The other commonly prescribed anti-androgen is called *cyproterone acetate* (Androcur). It is extremely effective in the majority of women, but also needs to be taken for at least one year for the full effect to be seen. Androcur is also very effective in the treatment of acne as well as hormonally induced excess body hair. It needs to be taken in combination with either oestrogen or the oral contraceptive pill. As it also acts as a progestogen, Androcur can be used as the progestogen component in hormone replacement therapy by post-menopausal women who also want treatment for hirsutism.

Various other anti-androgens have been used to treat hirsutism, but their use is limited by side effects and they are not more effective than available therapies.

Most women suffering moderate to severe hirsutism should be able to achieve an acceptable outcome using a combination of cosmetic and medical treatments. The therapy must be tailored to suit each individual woman's needs in order for there to be a satisfactory long-term result. Cosmetic measures are sufficient for a great number of women, but medical therapy is a valid option and should be discussed with the individual's physician.

For the majority of women drug treatment for hirsutism is only a temporary measure used to alleviate symptoms while a more long-term cosmetic program is established. Many young women find the lessening of their problem of excessive hair growth by drug therapy to be a tremendous relief and feel quite socially liberated when they are no longer inhibited by the embarrassment of their unwanted body hair. Often, after establishment of a strong personal relationship, or with the attainment of improved self-esteem, women elect to discontinue their drug treatment for hirsutism and continue the cosmetic management with which they feel most comfortable in the long term.

5
NATURAL THERAPIES

The general public and medical practitioners worldwide are becoming increasingly aware and accepting of the benefits of many aspects of natural therapies. There is essentially little difference between the *ideal* fundamental, therapeutic approach taken by both conventional doctors and natural therapists—treatment should always be of the individual, and prevention of illness is far better than treating an established disease. Experienced medical practitioners and natural therapists alike stress the importance of diet and lifestyle; however, natural therapists focus specifically on nutrition and frequently design diets which either emphasise a particular food combination, or eliminate certain undesirable foods (for example, the prescription of a diet high in plant oestrogens and calcium for postmenopausal women). Natural therapists aim to enhance the body's ability to fight disease and maximise natural healing using a variety of foods, vitamins, minerals and herbal medicines.

In terms of disease, natural therapies are not an alternative to conventional medical treatment, but they can be a useful support.

Natural therapies provide a gentle, long-term approach to disease prevention as well as alleviation of *some* symptoms. They can be dangerous if used inappropriately or prescribed by untrained practitioners who do not understand the potencies and toxicities of the remedies they are recommending. It is essential that anyone attending both a natural therapist and a doctor inform both practitioners of the different therapies being used. The two approaches are not mutually exclusive; however, failure to communicate could result in unwanted treatment interactions, or overexposure to certain compounds. For example, certain herbal products can have oestrogen-like actions and can lead to growth of uterine fibroids complicated by bleeding because of inappropriate, long-term use. If a doctor is not aware that a woman is taking this kind of herbal preparation, surgery may be recommended and performed; whereas if the woman tells her doctor of the herbal treatment, stopping the 'natural' medicine may enable the fibroid to regress and surgery to be prevented.

In the context of women's health, natural therapies using plant products can be divided into foods and herbs which contain oestrogen-like compounds, or *phytoestrogens*, and other herbal or plant medicines, or *phytomedicines*. For ease of presentation, I therefore use these two headings to discuss the application of herbal medicine in women's health, both in terms of disease prevention and symptom relief. Herbal medicine is the subject of much mysticism and myth. Many of the popularised herbal remedies in Western society, particularly the over-the-counter products, have no health benefits and are used at great expense to the consumer. However, I believe there is a role for the natural therapies in modern health care and have tried to present a rational and practical appraisal of the phytomedicines in common use for women.

PHYTO (PLANT) OESTROGENS—SOURCES AND USES

For nearly 2000 years, practitioners of traditional medicine have used plant medicines such as pomegranate seeds to alter reproduction in women. We now know that these seeds are a rich natural source of plant oestrogens and hence their medicinal value. Natural oestrogen-like compounds are widely distributed throughout the plant kingdom and are called 'phyto' oestrogens. When consumed by animals or humans, they have an oestrogen-like effect in the body which is much weaker than that of either human or synthetic oestrogen. There is increasing interest in the potential health benefits associated with consuming a diet high in phytoestrogens, and now many medical practitioners, as well as natural therapists and women's health groups, are encouraging women to include more plants rich in natural oestrogen-like compounds in their diet. Certainly, there is a great deal of evidence to support the positive effects of such diets; however, they must be viewed from a balanced perspective that includes consideration of possible health risks.

The biological activity of plant oestrogens was initially recognised by scientists over 50 years ago. An article by H.W. Bennets, E.T. Underwood and F.L. Shier first reported a condition called clover disease in sheep in the *Australian Veterinary Journal* in 1946. Sheep grazing on oestrogen-rich pastures were found to become infertile because their high plant oestrogen intake was interfering with their natural reproductive cycle. Subsequently, over 300 plants which potentially affect the reproductive function of livestock have been identified. The active components of all of these plants have not been established; however, of the identified compounds, the phytoestrogens known as *isoflavones* and *coumestans* are the most common.

Humans commonly consume a wide range of plants which are now known to contain phytoestrogens. In general, the more Westernised diet is quite spartan in terms of phytoestrogen content, in contrast to traditional Asian diets which are high in phytoestrogen-containing plants and plant products, the most well known being soy and soybeans. Those consuming diets rich in vegetable protein, and hence plant oestrogens, namely vegetarians and Asian populations, have a lower incidence of diseases such as heart disease, various cancers, diabetes and other so-called Western diseases. Clearly, various environmental and lifestyle factors and an individual's genetic make-up impact on the likelihood of these diseases developing; however, the importance of diet is a subject of increasing scientific scrutiny.

In terms of women's health, the incorporation of increased amounts of phytoestrogens in the diet is to be encouraged. Phytoestrogens may reduce menopausal symptoms and lower breast cancer risks. Nevertheless, although the consumption of natural oestrogens appears to be mostly associated with good health and disease prevention, excessive or inappropriate consumption may be detrimental and there are certainly some subclasses of phytoestrogens which should be avoided.

Table 1 True phytoestrogens

1	Isoflavones	Diadzein
		Genistein
		Formononetin
		Biochanin a
2	Coumestans	Coumestrol
3	Lignans	Enterolactone
		Enterodiol

What are phytoestrogens?

Phytoestrogens are naturally occurring oestrogens in plants which have a chemical structure and biological action similar to that of oestrogen produced by the human ovaries. Phytoestrogens appear to bind with the region of human cells where human oestrogens act (the oestrogen receptor) and may function either as very weak oestrogens or, under some conditions, as anti-oestrogens.

The oestrogenic potencies of various phytoestrogens are measured in terms of their actions on animals or their effects on different animal or human cell preparations. Different subclasses of phytoestrogens have been identified, the major ones being *lignans*, *isoflavones*, *coumestans* and the *resorcylic acid lactones* (see Table 1). These have all been found in animals, in blood or urine, and have been shown to be biologically active in animals and humans. Lignans, isoflavones and coumestans are true phytoestrogens in that they are found within either plants or their seeds. Their levels in plants vary according to the type of plant, its geographical location and whether or not it has been damaged by bacteria or insects. The resorcylic acid lactones are not true phytoestrogens but are produced by moulds which are common in the field and may flourish in badly stored grains. Classically, these mould oestrogens are detectable in animals and humans who eat contaminated cereals such as corn and maize.

It is somewhat difficult to compare the biological strength of the various phytoestrogens in humans. After being eaten, phytoestrogens undergo complex metabolism in the digestive tract. The way in which they are broken down and the extent to which they are absorbed depends greatly upon the kinds of bacteria which are present in the bowel, and this frequently varies between individuals. Other components of the diet, use of medications, particularly antibiotics, and other digestive factors determine what bowel bacteria are present and the way in which phytoestrogens are digested and absorbed. An example is the extent to which different people metabolise soy protein.

Soy protein has a high isoflavone content. Isoflavones are broken down in the body into a substance known as *equol*, which is then excreted in urine. The amount of equol detected in a person's urine is used as an indicator of the amount of phytoestrogen she is absorbing from her diet. Of a group of people who were fed 40 g of commercial soy protein daily as a substitute for meat, the majority had a 100 to 1000-fold increase in equol in their urine. However, some individuals in the group had little or no equol detected in their urine, indicating that they were unable to effectively absorb the phytoestrogens from the soy protein. In general, when compared with human oestrogen, coumestrol is the most potent phytoestrogen, followed by the various isoflavones: genistein, equol, diadzein, biochanin A and formononetin in declining order of potency (see Table 1). Of these, genistein has been the focus of most research.

Sources of phytoestrogens

A single plant can contain several different classes of phytoestrogens. For example, the soybean is rich in isoflavones whereas the soy sprout is mostly rich in coumestrol. Soy products are the primary food source of isoflavones, the family of phytoestrogens which have been studied most extensively. Coumestrol is more widely distributed, with fresh alfalfa and soybean sprouts having the highest coumestrol content (see Table 2). Soy products which have a high phytoestrogen content, particularly isoflavones, are now universally available in various forms (see page 81). Other significant plant sources of isoflavones include apples, cherries, potatoes, oats, garlic, hops as well as multiple animal fodders such as red clover, bluegrass and rye. Lignans are found in most cereals and vegetables, with linseed oil being one of the best sources. Food processing can result in the loss of phytoestrogens from food. Wheat, for example, loses much of its phytoestrogen component during modern milling processes. Some of the phytoestrogens lost by processing are mould products, which can have unwanted side effects and are best removed.

Table 2 Plants which contain coumestrol (ranked from highest to lowest content)

Alfalfa sprouts (fresh)
Soybean sprouts (fresh)
Soybeans (dry)
Green beans
Snow peas
Brussels sprouts
Dried red beans
Dried split peas
Spinach leaves

Beneficial effects of phytoestrogens

A typical Western diet is rich in protein and animal fat and poor in complex carbohydrate and fibre. Vegetarians, in contrast, consume less protein, total fat, saturated and monounsaturated fatty acids, cholesterol, and total calories and greater amounts of total fibre and grains. A wide range of health benefits are attributable to vegetarian style diets. These are partially a result of the elimination of saturated animal fat and the high fibre content of such diets, but we are now aware that the high phytoestrogen content positively affects health and reduces the risks of various diseases. Research indicates that phytoestrogens have a number of different biological activities in addition to their oestrogen-like effects.

Phytoestrogens have been found to have:

- use in the treatment of menopausal symptoms;
- heart disease prevention actions;
- anti-cancer properties;
- beneficial effects on osteoporosis;
- activities which protect against infections, i.e., anti-viral, anti-bacterial and anti-fungal actions.

Menopausal symptoms

In Asian countries like China and Singapore hot flushes are uncommon at menopause, being reported by only eighteen per cent and fourteen per cent of menopausal women respectively, compared to 70 to 80 per cent of European women. A high intake of soy has been associated with the low rate of menopausal symptoms, particularly hot flushes, in Asian women. Phytoestrogens consumed in the daily diet may act like oestrogens in postmenopausal women. An Australian study conducted by Dr Alice Murkies has demonstrated that dietary supplements with either soy or wheat flour (45 g daily) resulted in an average reduction in hot flushes by 40 per cent in women treated with soy flour and 25 per cent in those treated with wheat flour. The urinary excretion of phytoestrogens increased dramatically in the soy treated women, consistent with their high dietary phytoestrogen intake. The oestrogenic action of the soy flour was limited to reducing hot flushes. Vaginal cells were examined for oestrogen induced changes, but these were not detected. This is in contrast to standard menopausal oestrogen replacement which affects the vaginal cells, resulting in a healthier, more moist vaginal lining.

The reduction in hot flushes in the women treated with wheat flour was not surprising as wheat also contains phytoestrogens that are less potent and lost to some extent during the milling process. A much earlier American study has also reported that the use of a synthetic phytoestrogen based on a fungal phytoestrogen-like compound (resorcyclic acid lactone) was effective in the treatment of postmenopausal symptoms.

Further research into increasing the phytoestrogen content of the diet to minimise symptoms of the menopausal transition is clearly warranted. However, available data tells us that although a high phytoestrogen diet may lessen symptoms such as hot flushes, these will probably not completely resolve and many other symptoms will not improve at all. It must be appreciated that the differences between Asian and Western experiences of the menopause depend not on a single aspect of diet but on a whole lifestyle package in combination with cultural expectations. It would be a gross oversimplification to believe that differences in phytoestrogen intake alone account for fewer symptoms such as hot flushes in menopausal women in Asian countries. We know that women who exercise more, are less stressed and have a less negative attitude towards menopause are less likely to experience bothersome symptoms. Personal and community attitudes towards the menopause also have a major effect on the likelihood of an individual woman reporting symptoms.

For example, despite their highly phytoestrogenic diet, Japanese women continue to suffer *koune–ki jigoku* (menopausal hell). This is because the discussion of menopausal symptoms in male-dominated Japanese society is still considered a taboo, and the physical and psychological consequences are expected to be endured. The assumption that Japanese women do not commonly experience significant menopausal symptoms because of their lifestyle and diet is a myth which needs to be dispelled within Japanese society and the Western world.

In summary, although dietary phytoestrogens may confer considerable health benefits to menopausal women, and alleviate some menopausal symptoms, their full benefits should not be overestimated and may only truly be seen when consumed as foods, not extracts or tablets, and in the context of an overall healthy lifestyle.

Phytoestrogens and cardiovascular disease

In 1995, a review of 38 studies addressing the relationship between soy protein and cholesterol in humans was published in the *New England Journal of Medicine*. Overall, consumption of soy protein resulted in reductions in total and low density (LDL) cholesterol and triglycerides, but no change in high density (HDL) cholesterol was observed. People who had higher cholesterol levels to begin with had a greater improvement in their cholesterol and hence a greater benefit from eating soy. It is not definitively known whether the improvement in cholesterol with a soy enriched diet is due specifically to the phytoestrogen component or the amino acid pattern of the actual soy protein. It is certainly plausible that phytoestrogens could have an oestrogen-like effect on blood vessels and cholesterol metabolism similar to that of human oestrogen. It is well established that human oestrogens and those used for oestrogen replacement therapy not only lower cholesterol but also decrease the rate at which cholesterol is deposited in the arteries, and hence protect against cardio-vascular disease.

Soy protein, rich in soy oestrogens, lowers blood choles-terol levels in monkeys, whereas treatment of monkeys with soy protein from which the soy oestrogens have been removed has a minimal effect.

Such studies indicate that it is the phytoestrogen content of the soy protein which causes the lowering of cholesterol, and that although the oestrogenic action is weak, it is still significant. Although research is needed to further our un-derstanding of the beneficial effects of dietary soy on cholesterol, there is no doubt that a diet high in soy protein lowers cholesterol and probably is protective against heart disease.

Phytoestrogens and cancer

Phytoestrogens have been found to inhibit enzymes which are involved in the regulation of the human cell cycle, cell growth and cell transformation. The isoflavone genistein, the most well-researched phytoestrogen, has been found to exert a wide range of actions which potentially inhibit the development and growth of cancer cells.

Cancer cells can only multiply if they have a good blood supply. Thus an important factor in tumour growth is the ability of the cancer cells to stimulate the growth of new blood vessels so that the tumour can continue to receive nourishment and expand. Synthetically produced genistein blocks the cancer stimulated growth of new blood vessels. This inhibitory effect of genistein on blood vessel growth may be significant in terms of preventing cancer growth and possibly partially explain the lower rates of several cancers observed in Asian countries where soy is a major component of the diet, especially in Japan. Lower cancer rates are also seen in vegetarians and people who have a macrobiotic diet. It is not inconceivable that, in addition to using dietary soy products to prevent the development of cancer, purified genistein may be useful in the future treatment of established cancers because of its ability to block cancer blood vessel growth.

The consumption of soy products has been associated with a lower risk of breast cancer and an increased time of survival after breast cancer surgery. Both natural and synthetic lignans and isoflavones have been shown experimentally to inhibit the growth of human breast cancer cells. It has been suggested that the phytoestrogens block the more potent oestrogens produced by the human body by acting on the potential or developing cancer cells. Thus in terms of breast cancer prevention, the phytoestrogens may have an anti-oestrogen effect. In both Singapore and Japan, women who consume diets high in soy products have lower rates of breast cancer compared with other Singaporian and Japanese women who consume less soy.

A similar relationship between consumption of soy protein and cancer of the colon (bowel) has also been noted. People who have soybeans or bean curd at least once a week have a lower rate of rectal cancer. Various phytoestrogens have been shown to inhibit the growth of specific cells derived from colon cancers. The protective action of a high fibre diet may be partly attributable to the phytoestrogen content of the plant food which makes up the dietary fibre, although this is an unproven theory.

Despite the fact that some populations with high soy intakes have been found to have a reduced risk of endometrial cancer, other studies indicate that high levels of dietary phytoestrogens may increase the growth of uterine fibroids and this area clearly warrants further research. There have not been any reports of an association between phytoestrogens and increased endometrial cancer risk.

There is also a belief that phytoestrogens may protect men against cancer of the prostate by their oestrogen-like actions in the prostate gland. Again, populations such as

Japanese men, which have a low rate of prostate cancer, are known to have a high dietary phytoestrogen intake, mainly soy, in contrast to North American or Australian male populations which have both a high and increasing incidence of cancer of the prostate.

In summary, it is justifiable on the available evidence to conclude that the lower rate of cancer observed in individuals with a high soy and/or vegetarian diet may be, at least in part, attributable to the phytoestrogens they consume. However, this remains unproven. Again, it must be emphasised that it is as yet unclear to what extent the protective effects observed are due to soy and other phytoestrogens, and how much is due to the overall vegetable rich diet and exclusion of other processed or fatty foods.

Phytoestrogens and osteoporosis

Data regarding a protective effect of phytoestrogens against osteoporosis is scanty. Preliminary studies in both animals and humans indicate a potentially beneficial effect of both natural and synthetic phytoestrogens. However, further research needs to be conducted before any reliable conclusions can be made. Certainly, no detrimental effects of phytoestrogens on bones has been observed, and information to hand does infer that a protective effect of dietary phytoestrogens against bone loss is highly likely.

Safety of dietary phytoestrogens

The possibility of adverse effects must always be included in the consideration of any health or medicinal option in order to maintain a completely balanced perspective. The most available form of phytoestrogen is the soybean and its various products, which are consumed worldwide. Soybeans have been consumed by humans for centuries with no apparent adverse effects. Allergic reactions to soy products, although rare in adults, may occasionally occur in children. Concerns have been expressed that soy protein may affect the absorption of important dietary minerals such as iron, calcium and zinc; however, in a balanced mixed diet, this does not appear to be a problem.

Although most research has demonstrated beneficial effects of diets high in phytoestrogens, it is always wise to be cautious. At this stage it cannot be categorically said that switching to a high phytoestrogen diet has no risk. For example, coumestrol, the phytoestrogen found in the foods listed in Table 2, which is one of the most potent phytoestrogens, has been reported to promote rat mammary (breast) tumour growth in a manner similar to human and synthetic oestrogen. While coumestrol activity in rats may have no relevance to its activity in humans, such findings should remind us that the available information regarding the effects of plant oestrogens in humans is still incomplete.

Purified fungal oestrogens, which are not true phytoestrogens, have been shown to be effective in reducing menopausal symptoms. However, despite these beneficial effects there are concerns regarding the quantities of fungal oestrogens consumed by some communities, particularly in South Africa. The moulds that produce the resorcyclic acid lactones (fungal oestrogens) have been found in the past to contaminate not only maize and corn crops in South Africa but also have affected crops in Canada, the United States and Australia. Regular consumption of contaminated corn and maize over a long period has been associated with a higher rate of digestive and cervical cancer, although a cause and effect has not clearly been established. Such findings again reinforce the need for caution and restraint when dealing with phytoestrogens which otherwise appear to be simple, exciting and positive, potential modifiers of health.

Soy and soy products

Soybeans were one of the 'five sacred grains' of ancient China. There are countless varieties, the most commonly used being yellow and black beans. Fresh soybeans can be eaten after cooking for fifteen minutes in boiling water.

Dried raw soybeans need to be soaked overnight and then cooked in water for three hours before being added to soups, casseroles and other recipes.

Soy sprouts, which are rich in coumestrol, are eaten raw like other sprouts in salads and sandwiches.

Soy milk is now widely commercially available. Different products vary in taste according to the manufacturer. Some soy milks have a relatively high sodium (salt) content and, unlike cow's milk, do not normally contain significant amounts of calcium. So when buying soy milk to consume regularly, check the contents information carefully.

Soy sauce is made from fermented soybeans and salt. Ordinary soy sauce is very dark (shoyu or tamari) and very salty and is used sparingly as a seasoning or in marinades. Light soy sauce does not darken the colours of foods and thick soy sauce, which is rather sweet in taste, is usually used with fish.

Tofu or bean curd is an important soybean product made from curdled soy milk. It is rich in protein, vitamins, minerals and phytoestrogens and entirely cholesterol free. It is sold as either 'silk' tofu, which is soft and contains more whey, or 'cotton' tofu, which is firm and more suitable for stirfry recipes.

Miso is fermented soybean paste. It may be yellow to brown in colour, is very salty and is used in Japanese cooking for soups, dressings and sauces.

Tempeh is made from whole fermented soybeans made into cakes, which are sold in a dry form and must be soaked overnight before use. Tempeh is higher in fibre than tofu as it is made from the whole bean.

Soy flour, which is gluten free, is a Western-style soy product. As a phytoestrogen source it is usually added to drinks or breakfast cereal, but it can also be included in muffin and pancake recipes. It has limited use in baking as it inhibits the rising of cakes and bread.

OTHER PHYTOMEDICINAL HERBS IN MEDICINE

The word 'herb' has different meanings according to the context in which it is used. Strictly speaking, herbs are non-woody, seed-producing plants which die at the end of each growing season. 'Herbs' are also plants and seeds used to add flavour to cooking or for their scents. In the medicinal context, herbs are crude drugs of plant origin used to treat illness and to attain or maintain good health. *Phytomedicines* are plant medicines made in various ways from herbs. When used in a medicinal way herbs or phytomedicines are *drugs*, not nutritional supplements. The knowledge of the application of phytomedicines is based on centuries of practical experience. More recently, scientific interest in traditional medicine has resulted in validation of some of the traditional medical applications. Single herbs commonly contain multiple chemicals with complex actions. Therefore the appropriate use of natural phytomedicines requires an understanding of the actions of the specific herbs prescribed and respect for both their potential therapeutic and toxic effects. Phytomedicines are sometimes described as *dilute pharmaceuticals*. A classic example is willow bark, from which salicylate (aspirin) was first isolated. In order to achieve the equivalent recommended daily dose of salicylate to treat the average case of rheumatoid arthritis, it would be necessary to drink twenty litres of willow bark tea per day (a calculation based on a standard preparation of finely powdered, high quality willow bark). Willow bark also contains eight to twenty per cent tannin, and drinking a moderate amount of willow bark tea therefore results in consumption of an undesirable amount of tannin. In contrast, aspirin tablets contain only pure salicylate in a standardised dose form. The salicylate is of equal value, is equally natural and of the same chemical structure whether it be ingested as a pharmaceutical or as a dilute tea; so clearly, to achieve a therapeutic effect it is simpler to take a modern, salicylate, tablet formulation.

Natural therapies are not substitutes for conventional medicines for the treatment of major diseases such as infections, cancer, diabetes and so forth. However, many of the pharmaceuticals used to treat these diseases are derived from plant sources, for instance *digitalis* for heart disease from foxglove or the powerful chemotherapeutic agent *taxol* from the bark of the Pacific Yew. These drugs need to be administered in a conventional, medicinal form in order to provide a pure medicine in a specific dose and to avoid unwanted side effects. Taxol is one of the most promising anti-cancer drugs, especially for the treatment of ovarian and breast cancer. Unfortunately, its source, the Pacific Yew, is scarce, making the drug expensive as well as raising concerns about destroying large numbers of these trees. The recent availability of a synthetic form of taxol not only makes the drug more available to those who need it, but also protects the natural source. Thus synthetic does not always mean bad, just as natural does not always equal harmless and good.

As stated earlier, herbs and their phytomedicinal products such as teas and tinctures usually contain multiple active components. Occasionally this can be advantageous, and it is often said that the unique, natural balance of the mixed constituents of a single herb can protect against toxicity. We would be naive to believe that nature is always kind, however. Many herbs and phytomedicinals contain chemicals with undesirable activities, some of which can be quite toxic. Comfrey, for example, which has been used both externally to reduce wound swelling and ingested as a tonic, has resulted in several cases of poisoning.

Consumers must also be aware that, unlike prescribed pharmaceuticals which are stringently regulated, over-the-counter herbal medicines require no proof of efficacy or documentation of either short or long-term safety. They are also not required to be standardised in terms of purity or dose content. The processing of herbs into powders, capsules or tablets, therefore, is unfortunately prone to variation and substitution.

The analysis of 54 different gingseng products in the United States revealed that 25 per cent contained no chemical trace of gingseng. Similarly, not a single over-the-counter feverfew product sold in North America could be found to contain the known minimal amount of the active component of feverfew required for the treatment to be effective. Thus the quality, content and efficacy of many over-the-counter herbal products is highly questionable and the marketing of these natural remedies clearly requires greater regulation.

Natural therapists use herbal medicines as supportive therapies to enhance the body's own healing mechanisms. Treatment must be individualised to be effective and requires not only extensive knowledge by the natural therapist of the herbs used but also considerable commitment by the patient. Herbs vary in potency and quality according to their subspecies, growing conditions and harvest time. The effects of a particular phytomedicinal will depend on whether it is prepared from the whole plant, part of the plant or ground powder. Thus the establishment of a specific dose for a herbal remedy is often difficult because of the variation in the quality of different preparations.

Specific knowledge of the activities of many of the constituents of commonly used herbs is unfortunately still lacking and clinical research is incomplete. Thus natural therapists base their recommendations on a combination of scientifically founded information and tradition. Phytomedicines have been used by traditional cultures for hundreds of years to treat disorders of menstruation, infertility and menopausal symptoms. Treatment is directed towards alleviation of the symptoms rather than modifying the underlying pathological processes, and should always involve comprehensive nutritional assessment and advice.

Many women experience various symptoms which are attributed to their cyclical hormonal fluctuations. They are not symptoms of ill health, although sometimes the symptoms are significant enough to interfere with a woman's life. Premenstrual breast tenderness, or mastalgia, is a classic example. Some women have several days each month of tender swollen breasts which limits the clothes they wear, affects their activities, particularly sports involving any running, and may interfere with sexual relations. Although seemingly trivial, this recurrent symptom can be disruptive. It is a symptom of normal hormonal change, not disease. We do not know in scientific, biological terms the exact mechanism causing the problem—it may, in fact, vary somewhat between women. However, mastalgia is a common, recognisable and unpleasant symptom, one of many such menstrual cycle symptoms experienced by women. Traditional therapies in conjunction with dietary modification may improve some of these unpleasant symptoms; however, many natural remedies in common self-prescribed usage, particularly those popularised by the media, are often expensive and ineffective.

As emphasised earlier, herbs are dilute drugs, often with multiple active components. Thus, unlike drugs prescribed in conventional medicine, it is not appropriate to think in terms of using 'Herb A' for treatment of 'Condition B'. Herb A may have a number of clinical uses and may be an excellent therapy for one woman with menopausal symptoms but not for another because of the herb's different components and the women's different needs. Herbal medicine must be properly prescribed and cannot be considered an alternative or adjunct to more conventional medicine for the alleviation of symptoms without being so prescribed. Self-medication with expensive over-the-counter 'herbal' products is not recommended. It will more likely be ineffectual and can occasionally result in harmful side effects (as we will see in the section on Alfalfa).

The following discussion of various herbs commonly used for women is by no means complete or absolute. There is so much still to learn about female reproductive symptoms and treatment with both conventional and phytomedicines. In many instances—for example, in the treatment of PMS—the effect of both conventional and natural therapies depends primarily on the clinical experience of the medical or natural practitioner: this area of medicine relies heavily on the 'art' of practice rather than the science. Women seeking help and treatment need to be involved and patient. The 'quick-fix' is rare. All reproductive cycle symptoms are heightened by stress, poor general health, poor diet and lack of exercise and effective therapy and treatment, whether mainstream or alternative, must address these factors.

Herbs with oestrogen-like activity

Plants which contain compounds with oestrogen-like activity are:

- black cohosh
- alfalfa
- oatstraw
- squaw vine
- false unicorn root
- red clover

These plants do not contain true female sex hormones but compounds called *plant steroids* which have an oestrogen-like activity. They are called *phytoestrogenic herbs*. The phytoestrogen content of these herbs is low and their biological actions as oestrogens very weak when compared to the human oestrogens, oestradiol and oestrone. However, they can be effective in alleviating many symptoms of oestrogen insufficiency at the menopause and certain unpleasant symptoms associated with the menstrual cycle.

Black cohosh (cimicifuga racemosa) is also known as black snakeroot or cimicifuga. It is probably the most active herb in terms of oestrogenic effects and has been shown in several clinical studies to significantly reduce menopausal hot flushes. It has also been found to be beneficial in the treatment of PMS and painful menstruation (dysmenorrhoea). The effects of therapy are not immediate, with maximum improvement usually achieved after four to six weeks. The herb is usually prescribed as an alcoholic extract (one in one or one in two concentration) and, less commonly, as a decoction (i.e., the herb is boiled and then strained and the remaining liquid consumed). *Remifemin*® is a weak (one in ten extract) cimicifuga product that is sold as an over-the-counter remedy. Uncommonly, stomach upsets may occur as a side effect, but otherwise no major problems or complications have been reported with this herb. However, its long-term effects have not been studied and thus prolonged use is not recommended without professional supervision.

Black cohosh, appropriately prescribed, certainly appears to be one of the more effective herbal approaches to the management of menopausal symptoms.

Alfalfa provides a rich source of the potent phytoestrogen coumestrol and is widely available as a tea or in tablet and capsule forms. A remarkable number of different claims have been made in terms of its healing properties. Raw alfalfa is certainly an excellent source of fibre, plant protein, calcium and vitamins K and C. However, it should be consumed in moderation. Some commercial alfalfa tablet and capsule preparations have been found to have a very high coumestrol content, and the effect of taking such large amounts, especially for a long period, is not known. Coumestrol has been observed to promote tumour growth of chemically induced mammary tumours in rats in a manner similar to that of oestradiol and diethylstilboestrol (DES), reinforcing the need for caution. In humans, the consumption of large quantities of alfalfa seeds on a daily basis has been associated in a reversible drop in the production of blood cells (pancytopenia). Of greater concern, alfalfa tablets can activate clinically inactive systemic lupus erythematous (SLE) and must never be taken by sufferers of this condition.

Oatstraw is the green, leafy part of the plant from which oats are harvested and is a source of isoflavones, one of the classes of phytoestrogens. It is used as a prescription fluid extract by natural therapists in treatment of menopausal symptoms.

Squaw vine is less commonly used. Its properties are underresearched, although it is known to contain various saponins. It appears to have an oestrogen-promoting action which is not strictly derived from phytoestrogens, and again is prescribed as a fluid extract by herbalists.

False unicorn root also has been poorly researched. It is believed to contain steroidal saponins which have a direct action on the ovary and oestrogen-promoting effects. It is used mostly by natural therapists who specialise in gynaecological problems.

Red clover contains isoflavones and is prescribed for its phytoestrogenic activity, also most commonly as a fluid extract.

The ginsengs

Ginseng is the classic example of the inappropriate transfer of traditional Asian herbal medicine to Western society. It is sold commercially in a number of forms including teas, capsules, extracts, tablets, roots, chewing gum, cigarettes and candies. The composition of all of these products varies widely. In fact, an analysis of 50 ginseng products published in the British medical journal *The Lancet* found no trace of ginseng in some of the 'ginseng' products. Thus when buying ginseng over-the-counter there is no guarantee that what is claimed to be present is what you get!

The ginsengs are the dried root of several species of the *Panax* genus of plants, and have been used for centuries in Oriental medicine. According to the 'Doctrine of Signatures', an ancient belief by which the appearance of a plant determines its therapeutic value, the ginseng root is useful in the treatment of 'all man's afflictions' because of its similarity to the human form. Ginseng is extremely expensive, and the roots which most closely resemble the human shape can sell for thousands of dollars. Because quality root is expensive, substitution is unfortunately common. True Oriental ginseng is *Panax ginseng*, also known as *Panax schinseng*. The native American species is *Panax quinquefolius*, which has become so much in demand that it is now classified as an endangered species in the United States. Its commercial cultivation is limited as it is a slow growing plant, requiring specific growing conditions and takes six or more years to develop a saleable root. In Chinese herbalism the American species of ginseng is believed to be 'cold' and Oriental ginseng 'hot', thus the two subspecies can have different traditional clinical applications. Such subtleties are lost in the gross transfer of herbal remedies to the commercial marketplace. The active components of American and Oriental ginseng are various triterpenoid saponins known as *ginsengosides* (or *panaxosides*).

Oriental and American ginseng contain different types of ginsengosides, hence the difference in their subtle effects. It is not known in 'scientific' terms how the ginsengosides act in humans. Research has been limited by the lack of standardised ginseng preparations, and therefore difficulty in formulating a 'standard' dose to study, and the fundamental differences in the diagnostic and therapeutic approaches between Western and Oriental medicine. This is not to say that ginseng is not a valid therapeutic herb, but that it cannot be classified as a single pharmacological agent in Western medical terms. Thus its use cannot be simply transposed into the context of Western medicine for either research purposes or as a therapy.

Tienchi ginseng (also known as *san qui*) comes from the dried roots of *Panax pseudo-ginseng* and also contains some saponins identical to the ginsengosides found in the Oriental and American ginsengs. Although traditionally used as a 'tonic', it is also prescribed to prevent and treat coronary artery disease, with clinical research indicating a beneficial therapeutic effect when used for this purpose.

Siberian ginseng is not a species of *Panax* but commonly used in Russia as a cheap substitute for true ginseng. Its real name is *Eleuthero*, and it has been known to be misidentified and sold as a ginseng-based health tonic.

The traditional use of ginseng is as a supportive herb to induce and maintain good health. Ginseng is a potent stimulant, not a day-to-day tonic and not the kind of herb that should be sold over-the-counter. It is traditionally used specifically at times of 'low energy' and usually only prescribed for short periods, for example over two weeks, and not more frequently than twice a year. It has been reported to have oestrogenic properties; however, these claims have not been substantiated, and it is not traditionally used for these properties. Because of its strong stimulatory effect, ginseng should not be used by people who have elevated blood pressure or any acute illness, for example a viral illness with a fever. Some individuals are extremely sensitive to its effects and can experience overstimulation with palpitations, insomnia and diarrhoea.

Finally, ginseng represents the complexity and subtleties inherent in traditional Oriental herbal medicine. Its use cannot be simply transferred to health food shops in the Western world where its authenticity is questionable and its non-prescribed use cannot be recommended. It is a potent herb which has traditional, highly specific uses, yet in the context of Western medicine it remains an enigma.

Other herbs commonly used in the treatment of women

Dong quai, also known as *dang gui* or *tang kuei*, comes from the root of the Chinese plant *Angelica polymorpha*. Although well-known for its use in gynaecological disorders, it does, in fact, play only a limited role. It is known to contain various coumarin derivatives that can act as anti-spasmodics, which may explain its use in treating menstrual cramps. It also has some weak phytoestrogen activity and can be effective in the treatment of hot flushes associated with menopause in some individuals specifically identified by experienced natural therapists.

Chaste tree berry (*Vitex agnus-castus*) is native to the Mediterranean and is used by herbalists for female menstrual disorders. It appears to inhibit release of the hormone prolactin from the pituitary gland. It should not be administered to children, postmenopausal women or in conjunction with other hormones such as the oral contraceptive pill or oestrogen replacement therapy. Chaste tree berry preparations may result in increased menstrual flow and headache, the latter improving with a reduction in dose. It has been recognised for its value in the treatment of menstrual disorders by the German Commission E (part of the Federal Department of Health that reviews the safety and efficacy of herbs), and may be of benefit when prescribed and supervised by a trained natural therapist.

Sage (*Salvia officinalis*) belongs to the mint family and is widely used as a household remedy in Europe. It appears to be effective in lessening the sweating caused by a variety of conditions. This action has been attributed to the volatile oil present in the leaves. The volatile oil consists mainly of chemicals called *thujones*, which can have mind-altering effects similar to those which occur when smoking marijuana. The 136-proof alcoholic beverage absinthe contains thujones, and it is well known that very small amounts of absinthe can have disturbing and profound psychological effects. Vincent van Gogh regularly consumed absinthe, which is believed to have contributed to his psychological turmoil. Although some women find sage tea relieves their hot flushes, it should be consumed with caution, and long-term consumption cannot be recommended.

Raspberry leaves (See page 36.)

Evening primrose oil (EPO) has become one of the most popular women's over-the-counter health products of the 1990s. This oil, which is produced from the small seed of the native American wildflower *Oenothera biennis*, contains 70 per cent *cis*-linolenic acid, twelve per cent oleic acid and nine per cent *cis*-gamma-linolenic acid (GLA). GLA potentially can be metabolised to prostaglandins, which are important in the body's chemical reaction to inflammation. EPO is commonly recommended for the treatment of premenstrual syndrome, mastalgia and atopic eczema (dermatitis). The media, women and many medical practitioners appear to have become prematurely overenthusiastic about the potentially beneficial effects of EPO. A sound, prospective, randomised, double-blind (neither patient or doctor knows what is being taken) placebo-controlled trial of the effect of EPO in the treatment of PMS conducted in Queensland showed it to be no more effective than a placebo. Considering the evidence against the therapeutic benefits and the expense of this therapy it is hard to justify the use of EPO for either PMS or mastalgia. However, many women anecdotally report it to be of great benefit in alleviating hot flushes. There appears to be great individual variability in the effect of EPO on hot flushes and usually it is a matter of individual women discovering whether or not it works for them.

Blackcurrant oil (*Ribes nigrum*) and *borage seed oil* (*Borago officinalis*) contain fourteen to nineteen per cent and twenty to 26 per cent GLA respectively. Despite their high GLA content, neither of these oils have been shown to be effective in the treatment of PMS or mastalgia. Borage seed oil should not be consumed unless it is certified not to contain unsaturated pyrrolizidine alkaloids (UPAs), which are highly toxic to the liver.

Herbs with 'androgen-like' activity

Sarsaparilla is derived from the roots of several plants native to Central and South America of the genus *Smilax*. It is well known today as a flavouring agent, having been initially brought to Europe as a herb for the treatment of syphilis. We now know it has no such medicinal value. Most recently, it has been promoted as having androgen-like effects and recommended as an alternative to steroids to body builders. This also is in an invalid claim. Sarsaparilla does not have constituents with androgen-like activity, and should not be prescribed for this effect.

Yohimbe, the bark of *Pausinystabia yohimba Pierre*, has long been used as an aphrodisiac. Yohimbe contains a mixture of alkaloids, the main one called *yohimbine*. It acts by dilating the blood vessels, thereby increasing blood flow to the tissues. Small doses appear to enhance sexual arousal in animals, and it is possible that it may also have some central neurological actions. Yohimbe and yohimbine can cause some serious psychiatric problems, particularly if used by individuals with schizophrenia. It also acts as a monoamine oxidase inhibitor. This means that it will interact dangerously with foods which have a high tyrosine content (red wine, mature cheeses) and various other over-the-counter drugs. Although yohimbe *may* be therapeutically useful in the treatment of some forms of impotence, it is underresearched and potentially hazardous. It should not be self-prescribed.

No plant or herb is known to contain androgen-like compounds, despite claims that various different herbs have such properties. No equivalent to phytoestrogens has yet been identified for testosterone or other androgens. Herbs said to have aphrodisiac properties mostly act, if they do at all, via their overall stimulant effect, as in the case of ginseng.

LIFESTYLE APPROACHES

A dietary approach to disease prevention is a recognised and important aspect of mainstream medicine. Over the last two decades, awareness of the dangers of dietary fat and cholesterol has had some impact on the Western-style diet, although many continue to consume an inappropriately high fat, calorie dense diet.

If future research establishes beyond doubt that dietary phytoestrogens significantly reduce heart disease and cancer, the major challenge will be to successfully educate the general public about the advantages of foods such as soy products and vegetables and influence a significant number of people to modify their dietary habits. Further research is first needed to more solidly define the role of soy products in disease prevention.

For now, I certainly am encouraging women of all ages to include plenty of fresh vegetables and, if possible, soy products in their diets. Soy protein is an excellent, inexpensive meat substitute and, although somewhat bland, can be included in many standard recipes. Women still need to ensure that they are consuming adequate iron if they reduce their regular meat intake, and calcium if consuming less dairy produce. Again it must be emphasised that the beneficial effects of a traditional Asian-style diet cannot be seen in isolation. These diets are one aspect of an overall 'healthier' lifestyle, which includes being less sedentary and less obese, consuming less alcohol and probably being less stressed.

There is a great deal yet to be unravelled in terms of the qualities of medicinal herbs. In the meantime their potency should be respected and use of them judicious. It is wise to be wary of recommendations for the use of herbal remedies by people lacking specific training and hence understanding of these traditional medicines. Anyone seriously wishing to embark upon the use of herbal treatments for a specific condition, such as menopausal symptoms, should be under the care of a trained natural therapist.

Without doubt, we still have a great deal to learn not only about phytoestrogens and herbal therapies but also about the lifestyle approaches of other populations, particularly more traditional societies.

PREMATURE FAILURE OF THE OVARIES AND PREMATURE MENOPAUSE

Failure of the ovaries at a young age or early menopause is not a controversial topic as such, but one which receives little attention, is not often discussed and which has little written about it in the lay literature. Yet surprisingly, premature ovarian failure is common, affecting one in one hundred women, including young women in their teenage years and early twenties. If surgical removal of the ovaries before the age of 40 is included, the number of women affected by early ovarian failure is approximately seven out of every one hundred women, with considerable variation between different countries. This chapter involves a moderate degree of technical detail, but as there is little written on this subject elsewhere and since it is my experience in clinical practice that women with premature ovarian failure want to know as much as they can about their condition, I have decided to review this topic comprehensively.

Premature ovarian failure (POF) is the loss of the normal reproductive function of the ovaries in a woman less than 40 years of age. This means inability of the ovaries to produce adequate amounts of the sex hormones oestrogen, progesterone and testosterone, or to develop a mature egg for ovulation.

Most women experience the natural loss of ovarian reproductive function, the event we call menopause, between the ages of 45 and 55 years, with little variation in this figure between different countries and different ethnic groups. Women are often described as having an 'early' menopause when it occurs in their early forties and a 'late' menopause when the transition occurs in their mid-fifties. This age range reflects the individual variation in biological ageing of the ovaries between different women. Natural menopause is the inevitable end of reproductive capacity that affects all women. It occurs because the ovaries literally run out of eggs.

WHY DOES MENOPAUSE OCCUR AT ALL?

There is a decline in fertility with ageing in non-human female primates; however, menopause, or the total end to reproductive capacity in the middle of life, is virtually unique to human females. Evolutionary biologists believe menopause developed very early in human evolution, probably as long as 1.5 million years ago, as a result of natural selection, which favoured women who became prematurely infertile.

Human infants are totally helpless for the first few months of life and then continue on to many years of childhood dependence. In primitive society, women who lost their fertility at an earlier stage were not only protected from the increasing health risks of further pregnancies, nutritional deficiencies, exhaustion and risk of maternal death, but were able to fully devote themselves to the rearing of their highly dependent offspring. They were able to invest the maximum amount of time and effort in each new child and continue their commitment until each child reached adulthood. It is also believed that menopause may have played a major role in the development of human intelligence. The increasing childhood dependence of human offspring reflected increasing brain development during our evolution, and the prolonged years of necessary maternal care only became possible because fertility was lost, and women were thus available to devote themselves to their growing children, rather than additional births.

In the past menopause is believed to have occurred much earlier than it does now, probably around the age of 35 to 40 years. How is it then that the average age of menopause is now 51.5 years? It has been proposed that the limitation of female reproductive years, and therefore of childbearing, resulted in increased adult female survival, which further increased all human life expectancies because additional care was available to offspring. Over thousands of years of evolution menopause gradually occurred later in female adult life in the context of increasing human life expectancy.

In contrast to the evolutionary benefits of natural menopause and its occurrence now at approximately 51 years as a function of normal biological ageing in women, loss of ovarian function before the age of 40 is considered a premature event, even when it occurs for no clearly identifiable cause.

SYMPTOMS OF PREMATURE OVARIAN FAILURE

The age at which premature ovarian failure (POF) occurs depends on the underlying cause, if any, as well as the timing and rapidity of loss of ovarian function. POF occurring before puberty results in failure of sexual development and the absence of menstruation. Ovarian failure after puberty results in loss of menstruation after the establishment of apparently normal cycles in a young woman with normal sexual development. Some girls experience full sexual development followed by one or two menstrual cycles before the ovaries fail. Others, for example most patients with chromosomal defects, are sexually undeveloped and fail to menstruate at all, although there are a few girls who have a small amount of ovarian tissue which functions briefly, and who have some sexual development and a few menstrual cycles.

Girls who fail to enter puberty do not experience symptoms of oestrogen deficiency as exposure of the body to adult levels of oestrogen and subsequent oestrogen loss appear to be necessary for the development of such symptoms. Young women who develop POF after puberty frequently experience hot flushes, night sweats, fatigue and mood changes including emotional lability, irritability and depression. Vaginal dryness and discomfort with intercourse are also common features of oestrogen lack. Women with POF not only suffer from a lack of oestrogen and progesterone but also from testosterone, more commonly considered a 'male' hormone, which is produced by both the adrenal glands and the ovaries (see Chapter 9).

WHAT HAPPENS WHEN THE OVARIES FAIL?

The ovary is made up of incompletely developed eggs (germ cells) and specialised hormone producing cells lying in a supportive structure. The cells which produce oestrogen encase the developing eggs in numerous little nests. These cells are called *follicular cells* and the 'nests' are known as *follicles*. Ovarian failure is due to the extensive deterioration of these important follicular cells and the immature eggs (ova) within. Thus the necessary sex hormones can no longer be produced and fertilisable eggs can no longer develop. Blood levels of the important female sex hormones oestrogen and progesterone fall, and symptoms of oestrogen insufficiency develop.

The normal female before birth has ovaries containing approximately 7.5 million immature ova at the age of twenty weeks. By birth this number has fallen to two million and by puberty only about 300 000 remain. It is not understood why so many ova are necessary in the first place, or what determines their loss. We know that when the number of healthy ova reaches 25 000, usually at about 37 years of age, there is an accelerated loss, culminating in menopause at the average age of 51.5 years. When the rate at which the ova disappear is accelerated earlier, menopause will occur earlier.

Normally, the function of the ovaries is directed by the pituitary gland, which lies tucked under the middle of the brain and which sends hormonal signals to the ovaries. The pituitary, in turn, is controlled by the hypothalamus, which is part of the brain situated above the pituitary and which acts as the central control box for reproductive function. The pituitary produces the hormones FSH (follicle stimulating hormone) and LH (luteinising hormone), which act on the ovaries and stimulate the development of a mature egg each cycle and induce the release of the mature egg from the ovary by the process known as *ovulation*. When the health of the hormone producing cells of the ovaries, the follicular cells, deteriorates, oestrogen levels fall and this change is detected by both the hypothalamus and the pituitary gland. The pituitary gland responds by producing greater amounts of both FSH and LH in an attempt to switch the ovaries back on.

Therefore, women with ovarian failure have consistently very low blood levels of oestrogen and progesterone, and elevated levels of the pituitary hormones FSH and LH.

Women who have had their ovaries surgically removed also have the same increases in FSH and LH. This is because they are no longer able to produce sufficient oestrogen and so the pituitary produces more FSH and LH to stimulate the ovaries, even though they are no longer there.

There are multiple known causes for POF which are listed in Table 3. However, for the majority of women who experience POF after the age of twenty, an identifiable cause is rarely found. These women are said to have spontaneous premature ovarian failure.

Women are usually found to have POF after presenting to their doctor with loss of regular menstruation. This diagnosis has major life implications including loss of fertility and the short and long-term health consequences of oestrogen deficiency at a young age. Usually this diagnosis comes as a shock and women are confronted with suddenly having to reconsider their pre-existing life expectations and deal with the impact of their condition on current and future relationships. Women who experience early ovarian failure and the symptoms of oestrogen deficiency (see below), are different from other women of the same age who continue to have regular cycles, have normal levels of sex hormones and are fertile. Many affected women are sensitive to this difference and feel very isolated. They often have to deal with the physical, psychological and emotional aspects of their condition with little peer group support. Relationship issues emerge commonly as a result of POF. Men usually do not understand why their partners suddenly lack oestrogen, what the consequences of this are and how to deal with them. They feel uncertain and confused about issues like their partner's femininity and sexuality, yet these aspects are frequently not openly discussed. For some women, the ovarian failure and the loss of their fertility is the consequence of cancer therapy, either chemotherapy or radiotherapy, and although they try very hard to accept this as part of the cost of their recovery from their malignant disease, it is still a huge sacrifice.

It is important that affected women understand the nature and long-term consequences of POF. All women who experience POF require long-term hormone replacement therapy (HRT) in order to maintain good overall health. In addition to the loss of fertility, women with POF are at increased risk of developing premature atherosclerotic cardiovascular disease in midlife, as well as being at increased risk of osteoporotic fractures at an early age. The first 30 years of life are the most critical for bone formation and the achievement of maximal bone strength, therefore the earlier the loss of normal levels of ovarian hormones, the greater the risk of bone loss.

HRT in this instance is not a controversial issue and is not comparable to the use of HRT after the menopause. Women who experience early loss of ovarian function are oestrogen and progesterone deficient, and usually also testosterone deficient when compared to other normal women of the same age. Taking HRT for POF is no different from people with underactive thyroids taking thyroid hormone replacement or diabetics using insulin. Whether or not women with POF choose to continue using HRT beyond the average age of natural menopause is a different issue.

It is of great concern that not only do a number of women suffer symptoms for a very long time before a diagnosis is made, but also that it may then be several years before HRT is even offered to them. Again, this is particularly worrying in young girls who may lose the opportunity to achieve their ideal peak bone mass. Delay in diagnosis and treatment also wrongly subjects women to unnecessary symptoms, loss of sexual function and poor quality of life. Many women express anger that they have experienced flushes and fatigue for several years, but have been reassured that they have no physical illness. There is nothing more frustrating and depressing than feeling unwell but being told that the symptoms are due to stress, or just imagined or trivial.

Women and health professionals alike must be aware that prolonged intervals without menstruation are abnormal and must be investigated.

CAUSES OF PREMATURE OVARIAN FAILURE

Table 3 lists the principal causes of POF.

Spontaneous premature ovarian failure

It is estimated that five per cent of women whose periods stop unexpectedly before the age of 40 are possibly experiencing early ovarian failure in that they have high blood FSH and low oestrogen levels. This requires further investigation. Most women who are ultimately found to have premature ovarian failure have no discernible cause of this and are said to have spontaneous premature ovarian failure with normal chromosomes. It may be that such women have chromosomal abnormalities which are too subtle to be recognised, but when there are no accompanying abnormal health manifestations this is merely an academic point. Spontaneous POF is due to inexplicable early degeneration of the cells of the ovary. Some women who attend infertility programs are found to be in the developmental phase of spontaneous POF in that they continue to menstruate with rising blood FSH and declining oestrogen levels and are unable to conceive. Eventually such women go on to have an early menopause.

Table 3   Disorders causing premature ovarian failure

Spontaneous premature ovarian failure
Familial premature ovarian failure
Chromosomal abnormalities
Medical intervention
• surgery
• chemotherapy
• radiotherapy
Disorders of metabolism
• haemochromatosis
• galactosaemia
Infections
Autoimmune disease
'Resistant ovary' syndrome

It has been believed in the past that once spontaneous POF has occurred, loss of fertility is absolute. This is not always the case. Women with spontaneous POF commonly have a few healthy nests of eggs left in their ovaries, although they are immature and their numbers are insufficient to produce much in the way of sex hormones. Infrequently, one of these remaining eggs unpredictably responds to the stimulation of high blood FSH levels, oestrogen production switches on and the egg starts to develop. Why this can suddenly occur, sometimes years after the diagnosis of POF has been made, is not understood. In most instances when this happens the development of the egg is flawed and ovulation does not occur. Rarely, however, ovulation may happen spontaneously, usually in women with low levels of FSH. Thus the possibility of a pregnancy in young women suffering spontaneous POF is less remote than previously believed with a ten to fifteen per cent lifetime chance of conception. Successful pregnancy is usually limited to women taking hormone replacement therapy. This is because without hormones the lining of the uterus is undeveloped and unreceptive to a fertilised egg. Women taking hormone replacement are more likely to have a uterus with a suitable lining for implantation of a fertilised egg and an ongoing pregnancy. Blood levels of hormones are poor predictors of ovulation. However, ovulation and conception are more common in women with one or two FSH measurements below 40 iu/L. When FSH is found to be greater than 100 iu/L ovarian failure is probably permanent and irreversible.

Many women initially diagnosed as having spontaneous POF who go on to conceive are retrospectively given the modified diagnosis of 'resistant ovary' syndrome (see page 110).

Familial premature ovarian failure

The greatest predictor of the age at which a woman will experience menopause is the age at which her mother went through menopause. Therefore, it is not uncommon for women with premature ovarian failure with no clear cause to have a family history of premature menopause in either their mother or sister. Recent research indicates there is a gene localised to the long arm of the X chromosome which is responsible for some inherited cases of premature ovarian failure. This may be one of several possible genetic abnormalities which occur at random, or an inherited cause of POF. The identification of a specific genetic abnormality as the cause for POF in a family setting is usually only of academic interest. If the affected women are otherwise in good health, and suffer no other manifestations of their possible genetic variation, searching their DNA for a specific defect will not enhance their treatment or overall care.

Genetic causes of ovarian failure

Specific genetic defects are associated with impaired ovarian development and function of the ovaries in later life. Normal women have two X chromosomes. The genetic defects causing early ovarian failure usually involve an abnormality of the long arm of one of these X chromosomes. In the absence of two normal X chromosomes or critical material from one of the X chromosomes, the cells of the ovaries, which initially develop normally, undergo very early deterioration, often with complete degeneration before birth. The ovary is then replaced by a white, thin, fibrous streak and is known as a *streak gonad*.

The most common genetic abnormality causing POF is a condition known as Turner syndrome in which there is only one X chromosome instead of two. This is one of the most common chromosomal abnormalities. Short stature is the most frequent feature of Turner syndrome, but affected girls also frequently have heart or kidney abnormalities. A number of young women with Turner syndrome appear to enter puberty normally. However, it is more common for affected girls not to experience natural puberty and to need hormone replacement in order to develop adult female breasts and body hair. Again, this is a group of girls who also need HRT from a young age in order not to miss out on achieving their full bone strength.

There are also a number of other less common genetic conditions which are responsible for very early ovarian failure. Some young women with these conditions may menstruate for a time and even experience an apparently normal puberty before their ovaries fail in their teenage years or twenties. All women who experience POF before the age of 30 must have a blood test for chromosomal assessment. This is because in addition to having an abnormality in an X chromosome, a few women also have an inactive Y chromosome in their genetic material. The presence of a Y chromosome in this setting is associated with a substantial risk of future cancer of the undeveloped ovaries. All young women with POF due to a genetic abnormality with the presence of a Y chromosome must have their ovaries or ovary-like tissue surgically removed to eliminate their considerable risk of developing cancer. Since most cases of malignancies in genetically abnormal ovaries occur in women under twenty years of age, and such tumours are virtually unknown in women over 30 years of age, genetic assessment is considered unnecessary in women over 30.

As stated already, young women who have POF arising from an underlying genetic abnormality have varying degrees of pubertal development and may initially menstruate apparently normally. Therefore it should not be assumed that a genetic cause for ovarian failure can be excluded on the basis of normal sexual development.

Medical intervention

This is a common cause of the premature loss of ovarian function in women under 40 years. Treatments for life-threatening cancer such as chemotherapy and radiotherapy are often toxic to the ovaries, and obviously surgical removal of the ovaries results in an immediate surgical menopause.

Surgical menopause and endometriosis. When both ovaries are surgically removed by an operation known as *bilateral oophorectomy*, a woman experiences immediate menopause. In contrast to natural menopause the drop in hormone levels is precipitous and, untreated, women usually start to experience acute menopausal symptoms such as hot flushes and night sweats while still in hospital. The most common reason for the removal of both ovaries in younger women is extensive endometriosis involving the ovaries.

Endometriosis is a condition in which patches of tissue which resemble the lining of the uterus (endometrium) grow outside the uterus. These pockets of misplaced tissue most commonly grow around the ovaries but also can affect the surface of the uterus, bowel or bladder. Rarely, endometriosis can occur outside the pelvis. Classically, endometriosis causes heightened menstrual pain because the tissue reacts like the lining of the uterus at menstruation but as it is in the wrong place the bleeding results in pain. We do not know why this strange condition occurs. Various treatment alternatives exist, depending on whether the extent of the endometriosis is mild, moderate or severe, on the severity of any symptoms and whether fertility is of concern. In severe cases involving the ovaries, surgical removal may be necessary. However, before this is done women should first feel confident that they have tried all the appropriate non-surgical options. They must also be aware that, even after apparently complete and successful treatment, endometriosis can recur and long-term follow-up may be indicated.

For whatever indication, surgical removal of any ovarian tissue—for example, loss of part of an ovary when an ovarian cyst is removed at operation—will affect the age of menopause. Important variables include the amount of ovarian tissue removed and the age at which the surgery is performed. For example, it has been estimated that if one ovary is removed at the age of 30, menopause would be predicted to occur at the age of 44, assuming the remaining ovary is healthy. If the remaining ovary is abnormal, menopause would be probably even earlier.

Even hysterectomy alone, with the ovaries left intact, is associated with earlier menopause. It is not known exactly why this is so, but it has been proposed that the surgical procedure of hysterectomy disrupts the full blood supply to the ovaries and hence reduces the stock of ovarian follicles. Tubal ligation does not appear to affect ovarian function and therefore has not been consistently associated with early menopause, although there is the possibility of ovarian blood supply being disturbed if this procedure is carried out too vigorously. However, with an experienced surgeon, this should never be the case.

The effects of cancer therapy on the ovaries. With advances in cancer therapies, increasing numbers of girls and women who have been treated successfully for life-threatening, malignant disease are paying with the loss of their ovarian function and fertility. Drugs used in chemotherapy affect dividing cells, as found in the ovaries, with some drugs being more toxic to the ovaries than others. Younger women are more resistant to the toxic effects of chemotherapy agents on the ovaries as they have more undeveloped eggs. Some women stop ovulating immediately during or just following cancer therapy, whereas others experience a more gradual ovarian failure. The effect of chemotherapy is often only transient with some women having return of normal function of the ovaries spontaneously months to years after cancer treatment.

The ovaries are extremely sensitive to the effects of radiation. Again, the radiation dose which causes complete ovarian failure depends on the number of eggs present in the ovaries, which usually is determined by a woman's age. In women over the age of 40, a radiation dose to the ovary greater than 600 Rads will usually result in ovarian failure. In contrast, younger women who have had up to 3000 Rads to the pelvis have gone on to conceive. Radiation is more toxic to the ovaries than chemotherapy; therefore when the two treatments are combined, ovarian failure is more commonly due to the radiation exposure.

Metabolic diseases

Very uncommonly, the ovaries are affected by what are known as *metabolic* diseases. These are diseases in which certain substances accumulate in the body and damage healthy tissues. Examples include the diseases which result in iron overload such as haemochromatosis, or thalassaemia major, treated with multiple blood transfusions. Even more rarely, an inherited disease called galactosaemia, in which the sugar galactose accumulates and injures healthy cells, can cause POF.

Infections

Failure of development of the ovaries in a foetus so that the ovaries never function normally may rarely be the result of a viral infection in early foetal development. Female infants or girls affected in this way do not have normal looking ovaries but tissue described as *streak gonads*. They cannot produce ovarian sex hormones as gonadal streaks do not contain normal hormone producing cells. When gonadal streak tissue is identified, even when the cause is unknown, it must be surgically removed because of the inherent risk of cancer developing in this abnormal tissue. Mumps infection involving the ovaries is also a well known but extremely rare cause of POF.

Auto-immune diseases

Auto-immune diseases are a spectrum of conditions in which the cells which usually produce 'antibodies' and chemicals to fight infection and cancer inappropriately attack normal body tissues. Examples of common auto-immune diseases include insulin dependent diabetes (diabetes mellitus) in which the pancreas is the target of attack; thyroid disease resulting in either thyroid over or underactivity; adrenal gland failure, known also as Addison's disease; systemic lupus erythematous and several less common diseases. A link between premature ovarian failure and these other auto-immune diseases is well established. The frequency at which POF co-exists with other auto-immune diseases is somewhat variable; however, indicators of thyroid disease are frequently detected in the blood of women with POF. POF occurs in ten to twenty per cent of women with Addison's disease (adrenal gland failure). Some women with POF are found to have antibodies (attack chemicals) directed against the ovaries circulating in their blood. It is not known why these antibodies arise or how they interfere with the normal function of the ovaries. In summary, women with POF often have generalised activation of their immune system, implying that abnormalities in the immune system have a role in the development of POF in a proportion of cases.

'Resistant ovary' syndrome

The 'resistant ovary syndrome' is a rare condition in which the ovaries contain a number of eggs but are resistant to the stimulation of the pituitary hormones and so the pituitary produces greater quantities of FSH. It is not understood why the ovaries develop this resistance to hormonal stimulation. Although frequently mentioned, this condition is extremely rare, but the likelihood of fertility in affected women is low. An ovary biopsy (tissue sample) is necessary to confirm the diagnosis, but as this information neither changes the outcome or the management and can potentially damage healthy cells which are still in the ovaries, it is not recommended.

LONG-TERM CONSEQUENCES

Information regarding the long-term health consequences of POF is somewhat limited with most of the available data from studies of women who have had early surgical menopause. In this group bone loss is common and can occur rapidly as a result of oestrogen lack. Bone loss is of greatest concern in young women who experience POF before achieving their optimal peak bone mass. If oestrogen is not given, the bones will not develop adequately. Sometimes inadequate bone development can be missed when bone density studies are interpreted by people not familiar with the clinical problems of POF.

Early surgical menopause is known to double the risk of cardiovascular disease. Oestrogen is essential for the maintenance of a healthy cardiovascular system in young adults, both male and female. It is often forgotten that men have significant levels of circulating oestrogen, which are physiologically important. Studies of young women who have become oestrogen deficient as a result of medical therapy demonstrate deterioration in cardiac function which returns to normal when oestrogen levels are restored. The various actions of oestrogen on the cardiovascular system and blood fats are discussed in detail in Chapter 8. Fundamentally, prolonged oestrogen deficiency from a young age has a deleterious effect on the cardiovascular system.

Androgen deficiency in young women

Testosterone has important actions in women in terms of muscle and bone strength, energy levels and maintenance of sexual desire. Young women who undergo surgical removal of their ovaries abruptly lose their main source of oestrogen and a significant source of testosterone and are frequently distressed by their resulting lack of libido, which is not rectified by oestrogen therapy alone. Sexual difficulties are encountered by approximately 80 per cent of previously sexually active girls and women who have POF. Major sexual problems are associated with withdrawal from social activities, particularly in women under 25. Fatigue is another common symptom of sex hormone deficiency that is difficult to quantify and often attributed to other factors. Women feel completely at a loss, frustrated and misunderstood when they continue to feel dreadful, with chronic exhaustion and loss of sexual desire despite adequate oestrogen replacement.

Testosterone replacement frequently enhances energy levels and improves libido in young women with POF.

Women with POF secondary to or associated with other disease processes, such as those referred to already, will usually have other specific symptoms related to their underlying disease.

Apart from the experience of sex hormone deficiency symptoms most women with POF suffer anxieties related to their condition. Many have a sense of loss of their femininity and often their social life is adversely affected. A concern for appearances is common and young women frequently complain of dry hair and dry skin. Most women with POF who have not borne children naturally worry about their infertility, and this clearly impacts in a major way on their existing or future relationships.

Infertility

Infertility is probably the most dire consequence of premature ovarian failure. Not only is loss of the capacity to reproduce important psychologically but the irrevocable loss of ever reproducing is devastating for most women. Apart from the infrequent, unpredictable, spontaneous ovulation and conceptions that have occurred in women with spontaneous POF, the likelihood of fertility is remote, and for women with streak ovaries or surgical premature menopause, infertility is absolute. No therapies have been demonstrated to be effective in restoring fertility in women with POF. Disproven treatments include oestrogens, anti-oestrogens, gonadotrophin therapy and the drugs Danazol, Clomiphene citrate and Bromocriptine. Thus, any attempts to induce ovulation should be restricted to specific, controlled, clinical trials. Women with spontaneous POF who on the rare occasion ovulate and conceive can be reassured that the course and outcome of their pregnancy is no different from that of normal women of the same age.

The first report of a successful pregnancy with the delivery of a healthy baby in a woman with POF through oocyte (egg) donation was in 1984. Oocyte donation is a viable option for women with POF with pregnancy rates being reported by some groups to be as good or better than *in vitro* fertilisation. These rates vary between different infertility treatment centres and specific programs. Oocyte donation is a somewhat physically and emotionally demanding process as it involves monitoring egg development, egg retrieval from the donor, fertilisation outside the body (test tube fertilisation), implantation of the embryo into the women seeking the pregnancy and a receptive uterus for the implanted embryo. Women with POF need preliminary sex hormone therapy to prepare their uterus for implantation and then continued hormonal maintenance until the placenta is sufficiently developed to take over. In addition to the technical side of oocyte donation, the social, ethical and legal aspects of this therapy need to be considered. These issues are of major importance but are beyond the scope of this chapter.

DIAGNOSIS OF POF

All young women who fail to menstruate by the age of seventeen or who stop menstruating for a period greater than six months need to be thoroughly assessed in order to identify the underlying cause. There are several other causes for failure to ovulate and/or to menstruate ranging from abnormal gynaecological anatomy through to central brain dysfunction. It is often easier to divide women who stop menstruating into those who have adequate circulating oestrogen levels and those who are oestrogen deficient. Causes of not having periods but still making sufficient oestrogen, include rare abnormalities of the genital anatomy, polycystic ovarian syndrome (see page 62) and some forms of exercise-induced failure to ovulate, classically in competition swimmers (see page 53). Causes of failure to menstruate (amenorrhoea) associated with oestrogen deficiency are listed in Table 4.

Table 4 Causes of amenorrhoea with low oestrogen levels

Familial delayed puberty	• family history of 'late developers'
Premature ovarian failure	
Pituitary disease	• overproduction of prolactin
	• pituitary tumour
	• other rare causes
Central (hypothalamic) causes	• 'stress'
	• eating disorders such as anorexia nervosa or bulimia
	• continuous intense exercise
	• rapid weight loss
	• severe illness
	• psychological stress
	• international travel
	• poor nutrition
	• hereditary abnormal development of the hypothalamus (Kallman's syndrome)

Certain initial key investigations need to be performed to enable a preliminary diagnosis to be made. In premature ovarian failure, oestrogen levels are low and FSH and LH are elevated. Although uncommon, because some women undergo a transient loss of reproductive function, followed by return of normal ovarian activity, early failure of the ovaries *cannot* be diagnosed on a single blood test. A low oestrogen level with a concomitantly high FSH must be detected on at least three separate occasions, each at least one month apart, for a firm diagnosis to be made.

Approximately ten per cent of women who unexpectedly stop menstruating have elevated blood FSH levels and need further tests for possible POF, but many of these women will not be subsequently found to have this condition.

Chromosomal analysis is *mandatory* for all women experiencing ovarian failure before the age of 30 years.

Older women should discuss the option of chromosomal studies, as identification of an abnormality may influence other family members, sisters or daughters who carry the same defect in terms of planning pregnancies. Women of short stature, less than 160 cm tall, are more likely to have a chromosomal defect associated with their POF as there is a strong genetic link between height and ovarian function. When chromosomal abnormalities are found, the diagnosis of premature ovarian failure can be made with certainty.

Women who have a strong family history of related auto-immune diseases such as diabetes, thyroid disease or adrenal disease should have an auto-antibody screen performed to identify whether they are at risk of these associated diseases. This is done by having a single blood sample taken.

A pelvic ultrasound is often performed to assess the appearance of the ovaries and detect any developing eggs. Ideally, this should be performed using a vaginal ultrasound probe, which is less invasive than it sounds, since this technique results in the best pictures of the ovaries. However, when this is unacceptable—for example for a young girl or woman who has not been sexually active—an abdominal study will suffice. Ovarian activity identified by the presence of healthy cell nests in the ovaries is observed on ultrasound in up to 31 per cent of women with spontaneous POF.

If there is still concern that either streak gonads or ovaries with Y chromosomal material are present, the surgical procedures *laparoscopy* or *laparotomy* with removal of any abnormal tissue are essential to guard against the high risk of malignancy developing in these abnormal ovaries.

An ovarian biopsy to assist in the diagnosis of resistant ovary syndrome should not be performed, as the management of this condition is no different from other causes of POF, and the biopsy procedure itself may cause further damage to the ovaries of women who already have little chance of fertility.

TREATMENT OF PREMATURE OVARIAN FAILURE/PREMATURE MENOPAUSE

Any woman who suddenly discovers she has precocious loss of reproductive capacity requires a great deal of emotional and personal support. Infertility is often said to be the most damaging consequence of POF; however, the resulting threat to an individual's female identity is frequently underestimated. In societies where the ability to bear children is associated with womanhood, most women incapable of having children, as opposed to those choosing not to have children, feel very isolated and express feelings of inadequacy. Doctors deal very well with the management of the medical aspects of this condition, but are sometimes unable to relate to the sense of loss and the apparently 'irrational' feelings of incompleteness which torment some affected women. When the absence of ovarian function is predictable—for example in girls with Turner syndrome, or as the result of life-saving cancer therapy—infertility is commonly assumed to be accepted by the affected women, but in reality its loss is just as poignant.

Menopause support groups are increasingly common, and are a good initial point of contact for young women with POF. Such groups are also a good source of health information updates.

Having a healthy, low fat diet replete with calcium and regular exercise to stimulate bone formation and protect against cardiovascular disease is fundamental to the health and well-being of all women, but particularly important for sufferers of POF who, because of their early menopause, are at increased risk of bone loss and heart disease.

Healthy living is important and should always be encouraged, but there is an increasing tendency towards doing things 'naturally' associated with a reluctance to take prescription medications. This is an appropriate way of thinking for some aspects of ill health, for example losing weight, exercising and maintaining a low salt, low fat diet to treat high blood pressure or high cholesterol instead of taking tablets. However, lack of oestrogen during the adolescent and early years of adulthood is an *abnormal* state which constitutes oestrogen deficiency.

Oestrogen deficiency in young women is detrimental to their health and should be corrected. No 'natural' therapy (see Chapter 5) is a substitute for oestrogen replacement in a young woman. Plant oestrogens have limited activity in humans and do not appear to be sufficiently strong in their oestrogen effects to adequately replace oestrogen and protect the bones and cardiovascular system of young women. There is no analogy between premature ovarian failure and natural menopause occurring after the age of 45 years. The former is a pathological state that should be treated, the latter is a natural life transitional event for which women may or may not choose to use HRT and for which the natural therapies may result in adequate symptom relief.

Women with POF need to have a comfortable relationship with their treating physicians so as to be able to discuss the personal aspects of their condition and optimise their total care. Obviously, other specific manifestations of any underlying cause of POF need to be assessed and treated as indicated. Surgical menopause in a woman who has had previously normal sex hormone levels results in immediate and severe symptoms, which if appropriately anticipated can be prevented or at least minimised by starting HRT immediately following surgery. Young women who are sexually immature require initially very low dose sex hormone replacement that is only gradually increased in line with their overall rate of physical and psychological maturation, whereas sexually mature women with POF often need higher doses of oestrogen and progesterone from the start of therapy. It is vital that young women with POF are cared for by a physician experienced in this aspect of women's health.

Hormone replacement therapy is fundamental to the management of POF. Fortunately, there is now a vast number of options for sex hormone replacement including tablets, gels, creams, patches, vaginal rings, implants and hormone containing intra-uterine devices (IUD), so that an acceptable form of hormone replacement can be tailored to suit every individual. Oestrogen replacement will relieve the symptoms of oestrogen deficiency, restore and enhance sexuality, a facet so often neglected, and protect against the long-term risks of sex hormone deficiency from a young age. Women with a uterus also require progestogen replacement to prevent over-stimulation of the lining of the uterus (the endometrium) by oestrogen taken alone. Different women have varying sensitivities to the available oestrogen and progestogen preparations and frequently it is necessary for a woman to try several different preparations at different doses before finding a treatment program that suits. Women do not need to tolerate side effects of their HRT. Adjustments can always be made to therapy.

Treatment ideally should be with a 'natural' oestrogen which has the same chemical structure as the oestrogen produced by human ovaries. 'Synthetic' oestrogens, as contained in the oral contraceptive pill are best avoided for several reasons. OCPs will suppress the return of any spontaneous ovarian activity and therefore are not recommended for women with spontaneous POF who would welcome an unexpected pregnancy. Synthetic oestrogens such as *ethinyl oestradiol* and *stilboestrol* are incompletely metabolised and circulate as stable, potent oestrogens in the body. Therefore they are not appropriate for routine oestrogen replacement. There are also some concerns about the health risks in later life as a result of the very long-term use of OCPs in young women.

Young girls who have not been through puberty should start with very low dose oestrogen, taken alone for the first few months. The dose should be increased in six monthly increments so that sexual development progresses gradually.

Progestogen therapy is commenced for twelve days each month either when the first vaginal breakthrough bleed occurs or in the second year of oestrogen replacement. The gradual introduction of oestrogen minimises the likelihood of side effects like nausea, fluid retention and breast tenderness, and enables young women to psychologically adjust to their changing physical appearance as well as resulting in more complete breast development.

Women who have been lacking oestrogen for some time should also start with low dose replacement and gradually build up to their maintenance level, again to minimise side effects. Young women need greater amounts of sex hormones for adequate replacement than the standard doses prescribed for post-menopausal HRT, in order to match the blood levels of sex hormones for normal young women and to adequately build up and maintain healthy bones.

Androgen (testosterone) replacement can be extremely important and beneficial for women experiencing persistent fatigue, loss of well-being and depressed libido despite adequate oestrogen replacement. This is particularly common in women who have experienced premature surgical menopause. Androgen replacement also contributes to the development and maintenance of normal muscle mass and bone strength. When appropriately prescribed, masculinising side effects do not occur. This aspect of therapy is discussed in detail in Chapter 9.

I do not believe 'alternative' therapies have a primary role in the management of POF. Phytoestrogens (plant ostrogens) can be effective in alleviating symptoms of the natural menopause, but these are extremely weak, oestrogen-like compounds and will not provide adequate oestrogen supplementation for young women with complete failure of ovarian oestrogen production.

Women with POF need long-term medical care and follow-up. This is particularly important for girls with chromosomal disorders who need to make a smooth transition from paediatric to adult medical care. Women with POF need to understand the basis of their condition, the long-term health implications and the importance of their treatment. As for all health issues, the ultimate responsibility for good health rests with the individual.

7

BREAST CANCER

Breast cancer is the most common cancer in women in industrialised Western countries and the disease women fear most. It is a disease against which women feel powerless, which appears to develop unpredictably and insidiously, and which is globally on the increase.

It is the concept that this is a disease over which women have no control, particularly in terms of prevention, that mostly engenders the prevailing fear. Women dread breast cancer more than heart disease because they feel that it is a real threat to their life. But in reality, the ongoing risk of a healthy 50-year-old woman dying from heart disease is 31 per cent and the ongoing risk for the same woman dying of breast cancer is 2.8 per cent.

These are both diseases of increasing age, with breast cancer often the less lethal of the two when diagnosed early. Breast cancer most commonly develops in women over the age of 60, with the occurrence in women from 60 to 65 years of age being more than double that for women aged between 40 and 45. The number of cases of breast cancer diagnosed each year is increasing worldwide, but the reasons for this are not known. Clearly, genetic, environmental and lifestyle factors contribute to its development. Most women who develop breast cancer have none of the traditional 'risk' factors; however, lifestyle factors are now being recognised as having a major impact on breast cancer risk. An understanding of the significant environmental and lifestyle risk factors is the key to any possible preventative measures women can take to minimise their risk of developing this disease.

Less than 20 per cent of breast cancers occur in women who have a known family history (mother or sister) of this malignancy. The term 'risk factor' is frequently used by health professionals to help identify individuals at increased risk for a particular disease. However, being labelled 'at increased risk' can be quite anxiety provoking, particularly when the risk factor is hereditary and nothing can be done to change this. Therefore there are some important points which need to be made about risk factors in general.

RISK FACTORS

Risk factors are identified by statistical means using information from population studies. Identification of risk factors in individuals which increase their risk of a certain disease such as breast cancer should be used as a positive step in prevention, for example identifying the women who should have more frequent mammography. However, risk factors are less powerful predictors of the actual occurrence of a disease in an individual as each person's biological make-up is so varied and complex. Therefore labelling women 'at risk' can result in asymptomatic well women believing that they already have a disease developing. This should not be the case. Many women considered to have known risk factors for breast cancer never develop this condition. This fact should be borne in mind.

The anxiety about breast cancer among young women has been perpetuated by the media, but is not rational. Although breast cancer is the most commonly diagnosed cancer in women in both Australia and North America, it is less lethal than many other malignancies. In the United States, lung cancer is the leading cause of cancer death in women despite there being less than half the number of cases of lung cancer than breast cancer diagnosed each year. In Victoria the incidence of breast cancer is close to double that of bowel cancer in women, yet the number of deaths in women from bowel cancer each year nearly equals that from breast cancer.

More commonly, breast cancer is being detected at an early stage because of improved and more widespread mammographic screening. The smaller a breast tumour is at the time of diagnosis, the better the response to treatment and the better the prognosis. So even though breast cancer is the most common malignancy in women, if detected early, it is curable in the majority of cases.

Ongoing basic scientific research and large population studies are contributing to our understanding of cancer at a cell level and to increasing insight into the pattern of breast cancer occurrence in the community. It is essential that the community and government continue to support scientific research in order to enhance our ability to prevent breast cancer, diagnose it earlier and treat it more effectively. Transmission of the medical understanding of breast cancer to women in general is also vital so that women can be more aware of their own health risks and take appropriate preventative measures where possible.

Breast cancer, like cardiovascular disease, is a disease of modern, urbanised, Western society. The lifetime risk of developing breast cancer in North America is one woman in eight and in Australia one in fourteen; but in Japan, it is one in 40 and in India one in 50. This difference is not simply due to greater surveillance and diagnosis in some countries or to genetic characteristics, as Japanese women who emigrate to North America gradually acquire the greater risk rate of this region. Therefore lifestyle and environment have a major impact on the process of breast cancer development. There may be several things individual women can actively do in terms of lifestyle modification to decrease their risk of breast cancer or enhance their survival should it develop. As for the prevention of cardiovascular disease, measures to reduce breast cancer risk probably involve long-term, lifestyle modification. It is not as simple as not smoking to prevent lung cancer or being 'sun-safe' to minimise skin cancer risk however. Apart from inherited factors, the major risk for the development of breast cancer in later life is probably established during adolescence and the reproductive years and then modified by other environmental factors during adulthood.

WHAT CAUSES BREAST CANCER?

According to the Oxford Dictionary, cancer is a 'malignant tumour eating the part it is in, spreading indefinitely, and tending to recur when removed . . .' The medical definition is not quite so terrifying. Cancer is a term used to describe abnormal growth of cells which may result in the invasion of normal tissues with the possibility of spread to different organs, a process known as *metastasis*. Cancer is not a single disease. There are a large number of different forms of cancer with varying biological behaviour. The aggressiveness of a particular cancer is based on the propensity of the abnormal cells to divide and therefore invade or spread. The aggressiveness of a single cancer type, for example breast cancer, can vary enormously between individuals. It depends on the genetic characteristics of the cancer cells and the ability of the affected individual to combat the cancer.

Cancer cells are often described in terms of their degree of *differentiation*. *Well-differentiated* cancer cells retain many of the features of the normal cells among which they develop, whereas *undifferentiated* cancer cells bear little resemblance to the cells from which they have emerged and tend to behave more as a 'wild type'. For breast cancer, the tumour size and the degree of differentiation appear to be related. Smaller breast cancer tumours tend to be more well-differentiated and have a better prognosis. Women diagnosed as having a breast cancer less than one centimetre in diameter have a greater than 90 per cent survival up to at least fourteen years after diagnosis because these tumours are not only small, but are usually well-differentiated and therefore less aggressive in their growth and less likely to spread. All breast cancers arise in the milk ducts. Very early in their development, these tumours are called *ductal carcinomas in situ* or DCIS and by definition they are made up of abnormal cells which have not broken through the lining of the duct, that is they are not yet *invasive*. Ductal carcinomas in situ account for up to 30 per cent of the breast malignancies detected in some mammographic studies. They are too small to feel but are visible on mammography. Some leading breast cancer researchers believe it is misleading to actually classify these tumours as cancer because they are pre-invasive, and the main criterion for a tumour to be called cancer is for it to be invasive. There is great controversy now among breast cancer researchers, physicians and surgeons as to how these pre-invasive breast changes should be treated. In the absence of knowing which will progress to invasive breast cancer and which may remain unchanged is it prudent that all women with ductal carcinoma in situ be treated? Or are women with DCIS being overtreated such that some are having unnecessary breast surgery? How best to deal with DCIS is a major dilemma. It is a prime example of our increasing capacity to detect diseases at earlier stages, without knowing the significance of these early changes.

For example, we now know after extensive research that *dysplasia* (abnormal cells) of the cervix is a pre-malignant condition and that carcinoma in situ of the cervix, although pre-invasive, will ultimately progress to cervical cancer. Fortunately, when identified by Pap smear screening these early changes can be treated relatively non-invasively with diathermy, laser surgery or limited conventional surgery. In contrast, there are no equivalent non-intrusive ways of treating pre-invasive breast cancer, or DCIS. The most conservative treatment option is 'lumpectomy' in which a small lump of breast tissue containing the area of DCIS is removed. In some cases mastectomy (complete removal of the breast) is being performed for DCIS. Although it is confusing, it is important for women to be aware of what the uncertainties are in this area. With the increased refinement and availability of mammography the diagnosis of DCIS is becoming more common, and more women and their physicians are being confronted with the dilemma of selecting treatment while not yet knowing which treatment is most appropriate. Studies addressing the absolute risk of pre-invasive breast disease progressing to invasive cancer are urgently needed, but until such time as more definitive information is available, the treatment of DCIS remains in the grey area of medicine.

An important, unique feature of some breast cancer cells is their ability to respond to hormones because they have hormone *receptors* like normal breast cells. These receptors can be for oestrogen, progesterone or androgens. After a breast cancer is surgically removed the cancer tissue is examined for the presence of these receptors, and then classified as being oestrogen, progesterone or androgen receptor positive or negative. The presence of these receptors reflects the degree of differentiation or maturity of the cancer cells and this is extremely important in terms of prognosis. Having oestrogen receptors is a good prognostic feature independent of the size of the cancer at diagnosis. The significance of progesterone receptors is not completely clear. Progesterone receptor positive tumours appear to be more responsive to treatment with high dose progesterone, which is sometimes used as second line cancer therapy. Androgen receptors also appear to be associated with a good prognosis. Older women are more likely to have receptor positive tumours, so generally their prognosis is better on a population basis than for younger women.

The biology of breast cancer is complex and poorly understood. We do not know what trigger causes breast cells to become malignant. Cancers usually develop over many years. For breast cancer in general there appears to be a lag of ten to fifteen years from the first breast cell insult or change until invasive cancer develops. This is based on studies of the time interval between radiation exposure and breast cancer occurrence in women who have suffered excessive radiation, such as survivors of the atomic bomb in Japan.

For breast cancer to develop, some initial form of damage affects the central genetic controls of cell division resulting in uncontrolled growth of cells. This process is often termed 'breast tissue ageing' and probably occurs over many years.

The time interval between the start of menstruation (menarche) and the birth of a woman's first child is when breast tissues are most vulnerable. Breast growth and development begins with puberty, and although growth ceases when puberty is complete, the breast tissue does not become fully mature until the end of the first-full-term pregnancy. Therefore, the longer the gap between menarche and the first pregnancy, the greater the exposure of the cells of the immature breast to factors which can cause genetic damage.

The first full-term pregnancy has a major impact on breast cancer risk. Initially the risk of breast cancer increases for a time after the birth of the first child, after which it gradually decreases so that in the long term pregnancy has a *protective* effect against breast cancer. The effects of abortion prior to a full-term pregnancy are not known.

During a woman's first pregnancy, there is a burst of cell activity in the breast tissue with increased cell division and breast tissue growth. Any genetic damage or pre-cancerous change that may have occurred in the years before the first pregnancy is likely to be unleashed during this sudden burst of cell growth, increasing the possibility of malignant change. If this happens a cancer develops, which is then detected in the early years after the first birth. This is why there is an initial increase in breast cancer risk after the birth of the first child. However, by the end of the first full-term pregnancy the breast cells have matured and appear to be somewhat protected against additional cancer causing insults and more resistant to the effects of hormonal stimulation. The increase in breast cancer risk associated with a first pregnancy increases according to the length of time between the start of menstruation and the first birth. Therefore a woman who started having periods at the age of twelve who has her first child at the age of 35 is at greater risk of breast cancer than one whose periods started at sixteen and who delivered her first child at the age of 26. Therefore, during the childbearing years, breast cancer at a young age is more common in women with children than those without.

This temporary increase in breast cancer risk after a first pregnancy is not seen after subsequent pregnancies. In fact, additional full-term pregnancies appear to have a protective effect. In the long term, pregnancy protects against breast cancer. The cross-over from the initial adverse effect of a first pregnancy to the protective effect of pregnancy appears to occur after about fifteen years, so it is not until later in life that women with no children become more 'at risk'. Ultimately, early pregnancy and multiple births are each associated with a reduction in the incidence of breast cancer.

Other known risk factors for breast cancer such as *radiation* and *alcohol* have greater impact if the exposure or consumption occurs during the pivotal years between puberty and a woman's first pregnancy. The younger the age of exposure to either radiation or alcohol, the more adverse the effect and the greater the risk.

Childhood chest irradiation most commonly occurs as part of treatment for childhood malignancy. The vulnerability of the immature breasts to the carcinogenic effects of irradiation have been most clearly demonstrated among female survivors of the atomic bomb in Japan. The risk of subsequent breast cancer was found to be highest for the youngest girls exposed to radiation from the atomic bomb and decreased with increasing age. This reinforces the concept that the more immature the breast cells, the greater the effect of deleterious environmental factors.

Many studies have shown a clear link between alcohol consumption and breast cancer risk. The greater the amount of alcohol consumed, the greater the risk. Data from the Nurses Health Study (an ongoing population based study being conducted in the US) puts the risk of breast cancer for women who regularly drink more than one alcoholic drink per day at 2.5 times that of non-drinkers. This is actually a greater increase in risk than that observed for women with a family history of breast cancer. Elevated blood oestrogen levels have been demonstrated in women with a consistently high alcohol intake equivalent to three standard drinks per day, and animal studies have shown regular alcohol consumption depletes the liver of vitamin A. Women deficient in vitamin A are more at risk for breast cancer. Increases in blood oestrogen and lowered vitamin A levels are both plausible mechanisms by which alcohol may contribute to the development of breast cancer, but these are still unproven theories. The worrying link between moderate alcohol consumption and the incidence of breast cancer makes it difficult to recommend a safe limit for alcohol consumption for women. The association between alcohol and breast cancer risk is greatest for women who drink more before the age of 30 than at a later stage in life. The implication that drinking alcohol at a young age significantly increases future cancer risk warrants serious attention in terms of breast cancer prevention for young women.

Cigarette smoking has not been associated with breast cancer in most major studies; however, a link is apparent when the age at which women started smoking is taken into account. The greatest impact of cigarette smoking on breast cancer is a 70 to 80 per cent increase in risk for women who are heavy smokers, more than 25 cigarettes per day, who started smoking before the age of sixteen. This again ties in with the vulnerability of breast cells to environmental insults during adolescence.

What about women with a family history of breast cancer? There is a consistent increase in the risk of breast cancer among women with a mother or sister who have had this disease. However, the inherited genetic risk for breast cancer accounts for no more than ten to fifteen per cent of all breast cancer cases. A gene linked to breast cancer, BRCA1, has now been identified and cloned, enabling further research into the role of genetic factors in breast cancer. A variety of abnormalities of the BRCA1 gene have been detected in young women with breast cancer, but the frequency and importance of these variations are not as yet fully understood. A family history of breast cancer does not appear to be a good indicator of which women have an abnormal BRCA1 gene. Alternatively, the implications of finding out that a woman with no family history of breast cancer unexpectedly has an abnormal BRCA1 gene is not known. BRCA1 also appears to be a marker for other forms of malignancy, such as ovarian cancer. Currently widespread screening for abnormalities of the BRCA1 gene is not appropriate, and will not be until such time that the significance of an abnormal finding is understood, and guidelines for genetic counselling and the clinical care of women with BRCA1 gene mutation have been formulated.

The impact of a first pregnancy appears to be greater in women with a family history of breast cancer in that the initial increase in risk is greater and this adverse effect appears to persist beyond the menopause. This is consistent with the assumption that some women inherit genetic changes to the breast cells that are multiplied during breast tissue growth in the first pregnancy. Interestingly, the impact of alcohol on the risk of breast cancer has not been observed to be significant in women who have a family history of breast cancer.

From a hereditary perspective, breast cancer is linked to cancer of the ovary, bowel and endometrium. Therefore any woman who has a strong family history of any of these malignancies is at increased risk of developing any one of them herself.

OTHER FACTORS RELATED TO BREAST CANCER

Women who have had a cancer in one breast are more likely to develop a second cancer in the remaining breast tissue. Consistent with this general predisposition to breast cancer in certain women, specific changes detected by mammography (*dysplasia*) or by breast biopsy (*atypical hyperplasia*) indicate a two to three fold increase in future breast cancer risk. Any women with such changes must have ongoing frequent breast checks and mammograms.

Breast cancer has also been associated with exposure of the breast to the body's own oestrogen produced by the ovaries during a woman's normal reproductive life. Women who have an *early menarche* or *late menopause* have a longer reproductive phase and are at greater risk. An early menopause occurring either naturally or because of surgical removal of the ovaries, or a late menarche is protective against breast cancer, theoretically because the shorter reproductive phase results in fewer years of oestrogen production and therefore less hormonal breast stimulation. There is no evidence that oestrogen causes breast cancer, most probably it does not. Other factors cause the fundamental transition of normal breast cells to cancerous breast cells and oestrogen may act as a promoter of the continued growth of these abnormal cells—something akin to adding fertiliser (oestrogen) to a patch of weeds (cancer cells). Oestrogen alone increases breast cell division, but oestrogen and progesterone together induce more. During breast feeding the levels of oestrogen and progesterone are reduced, and breast feeding, particularly at a young age, appears to be protective against breast cancer. The evidence for this has been somewhat inconsistent, most probably because the total length of time most Westernised women breastfeed is relatively brief. A protective effect may require several pregnancies, each followed by breastfeeding for a prolonged period. Women in the US who breastfeed for a total of more than 24 months

are at a slightly reduced risk of breast cancer in the premenopausal years; however, breastfeeding has not been shown to
protect against post-menopausal breast cancer. In contrast,
studies in China where more than half the women breastfeed
for at least three years indicate long-term lactation protects
against both pre-menopausal and post-menopausal breast
cancer.

Until recently, use of the *oral contraceptive pill* was not
believed to influence the probability of developing breast
cancer. There is now some evidence of a possible association
between increased risk and the long-term use of combined
oestrogen and progestogen containing oral contraceptives,
particularly in women who take the pill for four or more
years before their first pregnancy. However, the information
is incomplete and should not be a cause for individual concern
at this stage. Currently, studies addressing the relationship
between OCP use and breast cancer are being conducted and
we must await their outcome before further conclusions can
be made.

Dietary factors have been the focus of much research in
relation to breast cancer. Food, which we all take for granted,
is, in fact, chemically daunting. Fruit and vegetables contain
multiple chemicals with complex interactions, some of which
inhibit cancer growth, as well as natural toxins which can be
cancer promoting. So much is said and written about the pros
and cons of a whole variety of foods that it is often difficult
to pick our way through the maze of food faddism, hype and
occasional charlatanism. The nutritional supplement industry,
encompassing vitamins, minerals and 'natural' supplements,
is big business, relying on the vulnerability of health conscious
consumers. For example, the antioxidant vitamins C, E and
beta carotene are probably important for the body's defence
against molecules called free radicals, which are generated in
the course of normal metabolism. These vitamins occur in
abundance in fresh fruit and vegetables. Research has shown
that large intakes of vitamins C or E as supplements do not

protect against breast cancer, whereas women who have at least moderate intakes of vitamins A, C and E as part of their food do appear to be less likely to develop breast cancer. It appears that the various chemical components found in vegetables act together and reduce breast cancer risk. Vitamin tablets are not a substitute for healthy food.

A low intake of vitamin A has been associated with increased breast cancer risk, but the benefit of vitamin A supplements may be limited to women with an otherwise inadequate vitamin A intake.

A predominantly vegetarian diet does appear to protect against breast cancer. There are several reasons why this is so. Firstly, there are the benefits of exclusion. People who eat mostly grains, fruit and vegetables don't tend to eat junk food or highly processed or fatty food, and avoidance of these foods may be protective. Furthermore, vegetarians usually consume fewer calories per day by excluding meat and cheese which are relatively calorie dense foods. *Calorie restriction* is one of the most effective ways of reducing the incidence of cancer in laboratory animals. It appears that in the long term consuming only a modest diet in terms of energy content may lower the risk of cancer, and the difference in calorie intake between undeveloped countries and the Western world may be one of the factors observed contributing to the different cancer rates, including breast cancer. It has been hypothesised that women who have a higher fat intake are at greater risk for breast cancer. However, there is no evidence that limiting dietary fat will reduce breast cancer risk.

Women who consume a diet *high in fibre*, greater than 28 grams of fibre each day, have a lower rate of breast cancer than women who regularly eat less fibre, under fourteen grams daily. Foods high in fibre include fruit (four to five grams per piece); muesli (an average of five grams per serve); vegetables (usually four grams per serve); and wholemeal bread (about three grams per slice). High fibre in the diet binds oestrogen, which is contained in bile in the gut, and prevents it from being reabsorbed. Instead it is excreted in the faeces. Therefore high dietary fibre prevents the body's own oestrogen from being 'recycled' and reduces a woman's exposure to her own hormones.

Diets high in fibre also have a high *phytoestrogen* content, which independently appears to exert a protective effect against breast cancer. Phytoestrogens are substances found in some plants and soy products which have oestrogen-like activity (see Chapter 5).

Cruciferous (flower-like) vegetables such as broccoli, cabbage and brussels sprouts contain chemical compounds which may have anti-cancer actions. Some scientists believe the plant chemicals contained in these vegetables can influence the way oestrogen is metabolised in the body and hence have an anti-breast cancer effect.

Clearly, fresh vegetables contain multiple, diverse, chemical compounds which contribute to good health and appear to have some anti-cancer actions. The analysis of these plant chemicals and their effects is far from complete. The way in which a vegetarian diet specifically protects against breast cancer is not fully understood, but again the protective effect appears genuine. Nutritional supplements such as multi or mega-dose vitamins are no substitute for eating real vegetables as the complexities and subtleties of the chemicals in plants cannot be reduced to a simple pill.

The role of *environmental oestrogen-like compounds* in breast cancer development is controversial. These compounds have been termed *xenoestrogens* (foreign oestrogens) and include oestrogen-like chemicals found in various insecticides such as DDT, which is now banned, plastics and aromatic hydrocarbons in petroleum. It must be emphasised that the associations between these compounds and breast cancer are highly speculative, but the available data is provocative enough to warrant further research into the possibility of a link. *Chronic stress* is known to lower the body's defences.

Some studies have implicated a link between stress and breast cancer development and others have been inconclusive. Most recent evidence does not support a relationship between stressful life events and the development of breast cancer.

WHY IS THE INCIDENCE OF BREAST CANCER INCREASING?

The reported incidence of breast cancer has risen steadily worldwide over the past few decades as we have altered the way we live. Breast cancer is more common in industrialised nations but is also increasing in some developing countries, particularly in areas of previous low incidence such as Asia. Certainly improved detection contributes to an apparent increase in breast cancer, but with ongoing screening this is not sustained.

The changes that have occurred in reproductive parameters in women over the last decade as a result of lifestyle changes have a major impact on breast cancer rates. As a result of improved nutrition, less childhood illness and possibly less physical activity, the average age of menarche has decreased from sixteen to less than thirteen, over the last century. Simultaneously, the average age at which women deliver their first child has increased, resulting in prolongation of the vulnerable years between puberty and breast maturation which occurs with the first pregnancy. Also, the number of children born to each woman has decreased, along with changes in breastfeeding patterns, particularly in the duration of breastfeeding. As stated earlier, delayed first pregnancy, fewer children and short duration of breastfeeding all contribute to increased breast cancer rates. Adult height, probably reflecting improved childhood and adolescent nutrition, also correlates with the international rates of breast cancer, and has been observed to be a strong predictor of breast cancer risk for post-menopausal women.

In most populations height has increased over the last century, reflecting improved nutrition. Overall dietary patterns have changed considerably, especially in the past 50 years, and variations in both the calorie content and plant-product content between developed and undeveloped nations has a major impact on the populations of different countries. Western women today are more likely to smoke during adolescence, exercise little and drink alcohol than their counterparts in less developed nations, or women of their own country 50 years ago.

The contribution of negative lifestyle factors to the risk of breast cancer is very significant, but generally poorly acknowledged. I believe these differences in lifestyle and environments are almost certainly the main cause for differences in observed breast cancer rates between populations of women. Breast cancer rates rise with increasing Westernisation and urbanisation, and, without doubt, recognition of this pattern is one of the keys to the prevention of this malignancy.

HORMONE REPLACEMENT THERAPY AND BREAST CANCER

The issue of hormone replacement therapy (HRT) and breast cancer has become inappropriately controversial and unnecessarily polarised. Not only is the general public confused but the majority of medical practitioners are overwhelmed by the opposing views and conflicting data. There has also been a great deal of irresponsible, alarmist reporting by the media concerning HRT and breast cancer, which has resulted in the widespread dissemination of inaccurate information. Media reports of increases in risk of breast cancer with HRT have been imbalanced and thus irresponsible, as only the risks are highlighted with no reference to the benefits. A balanced perspective can only be achieved by being emotionally detached and conversant with both the recent and past medical literature addressing the topic of HRT and breast cancer. All the studies dealing with the interaction between HRT and breast cancer have been either far too small or in some way flawed so that to date there are *no* conclusive data. The major studies have involved women who have themselves chosen whether or not to take post-menopausal oestrogen before entering the studies. This means that the women have self-selected their treatment resulting in 'selection-bias', which then influences the outcomes. For example, women who choose to use HRT are more likely to have had no or few children, and if the latter to have had children after the age of 30; consume alcohol; have a past history of benign breast disease; live in cities and be of higher socio-economic status. These are all known risk factors for breast cancer and therefore, as a group, women who use post-menopausal oes-trogen have a high-risk breast cancer profile. Even though researchers have used sophisticated statistical means to try to eliminate these biases, the available data must be viewed with some reservation. The situation is further complicated by the fact that breast cancer is not only the most common cancer in women but also most frequently affects women over the age of 50, and most women using HRT are in this age group. When breast cancer occurs in a woman over 50 years taking HRT, it should not immediately be assumed that HRT is the cause.

Furthermore, to date, all the studies addressing post-menopausal oestrogen use involve women taking oestrogen tablets, mostly *conjugated equine oestrogen* (Premarin). There is a paucity of information available regarding the use of other types of oestrogen tablets, oestrogen patches or implants and breast cancer risk.

The greatest bodies of information concerning oestrogen use and breast cancer have been generated in the US. Unfor-tunately, the results from these major studies have generally been over-interpreted and wrongly believed to be equally applicable to women living in other countries. A report from the American Nurses Health Study published in the *New England Journal of Medicine* in June 1995 is a classic example. The Nurses Health Study was established in 1976 when 121 700 American female registered nurses, 30 to 55 years of age, completed a mailed health questionnaire. Subsequent analysis of data derived from this ongoing study has greatly contributed to our understanding of women's health. However, this data should not be interpreted out of context, but be seen for what it truly represents. The underlying incidence of breast cancer in American women exceeds that of any other country, and thus the women in this study are already at greater risk for breast cancer than, for example, Australian women. We cannot therefore assume that the effect of oestrogen therapy on the American nurses who are at baseline a higher risk group is translatable to Australian women. The prescribing patterns between the two countries have also been very different over the last two decades. Most of the women in this study only took oestrogen for three out of every four weeks, whereas in Australia it has been taken continuously for many years. Progestogens were less often prescribed along with oestrogen in the US in the early 1980s, but over the years this has become more commonplace. Nearly all the progestogen used by the women was for fourteen days or less per month. In contrast, in Australia many women take their progestogen continuously. The effects of hormones on breast cells can be quite different when the hormones are given intermittently as opposed to continuously. Therefore as the manner in which HRT was mostly prescribed in this study is so different, against a background of different underlying breast cancer rates between the two countries, the conclusions from this and other American studies cannot be generalised to include women from other nations such as Australia. The authors concluded from the recent analysis of the Nurses Health Study data that there was an observed elevated risk of invasive breast cancer among women who were current users of either oestrogen alone or oestrogen plus progesterone. The increase in risk was said to be greatest for women older than 55 who had used HRT for five or more years. However, it was also stated that 'the small number of cases (of breast cancer) among women taking estrogen plus progestin preclude detailed analysis of the risk (of taking progesterone as part of an HRT regimen) according to duration of use and age.' Since in Australia, and now increasingly in the US, oestrogen is usually prescribed in conjunction with progesterone, this aspect of the data generated from the Nurses Health Study is possibly totally meaningless. Yet the publication of this study and its subsequent reporting in the media has had a huge international impact. The inappropriateness of this was neither the fault nor the responsibility of the authors who reported their data accurately and clearly, but due to glib extrapolation and distortion of their data by the media.

In contrast to the hype over the Nurses Health Study report, the media chose to ignore the publication of the King County, Washington State, HRT and Breast Cancer Study reported in the *Journal of the American Medical Association* one month later. This was a population-based, case-controlled study of women aged 50 to 64 who had breast cancer. This means that women with breast cancer in the population were identified, and their use of oestrogens and progestogens were compared with age-matched women selected at random from the community. This large population-based study of middle-aged women found no overall association between breast cancer risk and the use of post-menopausal hormone therapy. Nor was there any association between extended duration of oestrogen use, greater than twenty years, and breast cancer. Compared with women who had not used post-menopausal HRT in this study, those who had taken oestrogen and progestogen for eight or more years were observed to have a 60 per cent reduction in breast cancer risk.

So what does all this mean? Over the timeframe of both of these studies, prescribing practices for HRT have changed. The use of combined oestrogen-progestogen HRT has only recently become prevalent in the US, and the use of continuous progestogen is only just becoming popular. There is no available data that assesses the current way HRT is prescribed and breast cancer risk. Available data indicates that progesterone taken for twelve to fourteen days each month is not protective against breast cancer. There is some preliminary evidence that progestogen given continuously with oestrogen may not result in an increase in breast cancer risk and may even offer some protection for the breast.

Most of the studies dealing with HRT and breast cancer look at the *incidence* of breast cancer with no information regarding overall *mortality*. Given the cardiovascular-protective effects of oestrogen and that post-menopausal oestrogen use reduces the incidence of stroke and heart attacks, the mortality from all causes may be reduced by twenty per cent or more among current users of HRT even though the risk of breast cancer may be elevated. Therefore for women with risk factors for heart disease, osteoporosis or dementia, the benefits of post-menopausal oestrogen are likely to far outweigh any possible increase in breast cancer risk. In perspective, the increase in breast cancer risk with HRT observed in the most negative study is still significantly less than the increase in risk observed with moderate regular alcohol consumption.

Importantly, any increase in risk associated with current use of post-menopausal hormones does not differ between women with and without a family history of breast cancer. Although medical practitioners and women with a family history of breast cancer prefer to avoid post-menopausal HRT, there is no scientific data to justify this caution. Women with a family history of breast cancer who suffer with menopausal symptoms and who are fully informed about the pros and cons of treatment should not be denied HRT if they wish to take it, and should participate in a long-term breast cancer surveillance program irrespective of whether or not they take oestrogen.

The 1990s debate regarding breast cancer and HRT may soon become redundant with the development of a new class of drugs known as *Selective Estrogen Receptor Modulators*, or SERMs. These novel compounds demonstrate the ability to act like oestrogen in some parts of the body, while opposing the actions of oestrogen in other tissues. Tamoxifen, which was originally developed as an anti-oestrogen to treat breast cancer, has been found to act like oestrogen in bone and prevent bone loss, and lower cholesterol levels. However, like oestrogen, tamoxifen stimulates the lining of the uterus and may increase the risk of endometrial cancer. Raloxifene is a newer drug of this class which acts as an anti-oestrogen in the breast. It appears to have little or no stimulating effect on the uterus, but, like oestrogen, prevents bone loss and lowers blood cholesterol levels in an oestrogen-like manner. Such new drugs with selective beneficial oestrogen-like effects on bone and blood cholesterol may prove to be important alternatives to traditional post-menopausal oestrogen replacement in the near future. Extensive clinical studies are still required to establish the effects of these drugs on the common menopausal symptoms like hot flushes, mood and sexuality, their long-term benefits for bone and the cardiovascular system, but, most importantly, their safety.

In conclusion, an individual's decision whether or not to use HRT depends on the severity of her symptoms as judged by herself and not by others, and her personal needs and expectations. The impact of the use of HRT on breast cancer is relatively minor in comparison with the far more significant impact of Western lifestyle on the increasing frequency of this disease—and it's a matter of keeping all of what we know in perspective.

SCREENING AND DETECTION OF BREAST CANCER

As we have seen breast cancer rates over the last few decades have been increasing, but between 1989 and 1992 the death rate in North American white women actually declined and this has been largely attributed to increased screening and therefore earlier detection. Early diagnosis of breast cancer has a profound effect on survival.

Women aged twenty and over are advised to conduct monthly breast self-examination (BSE). By familiarising herself with the texture of her own breast a woman can more readily detect any change. BSE pamphlets are available in most family doctors' practices, and doctors can further explain the method of BSE. Asymptomatic women should have their breasts examined by a trained health professional every three years up until the age of 40 and annually thereafter.

Mammography is a simple, low dose X-ray procedure used to detect abnormalities in breast tissue. Screening mammography is performed on asymptomatic women who have apparently normal breasts. Mammography is aimed at detecting breast cancer before it can be felt. Like all investigatory procedures it is not perfect and up to ten per cent of breast cancers may initially go undetected, hence the importance of combining repeated mammographic screening with regular breast self-examination. All women over the age of 50 should have a screening mammogram performed every two years. Routine screening mammography is not generally recommended for women between the ages of 40 and 49; however, this is to some degree controversial. Younger women have more dense breast tissue than post-menopausal women and screening in this younger age group does sometimes present difficulties with interpretation. Most recently, good evidence indicates that screening mammography in women aged 40 to 49 significantly reduces the death rate from breast cancer, and thus I believe screening mammography for all women over the age of 40 should be recommended.

Younger women at increased risk of breast cancer, that is having a mother or sister with breast cancer, or other specific indications, may be individually advised to have screening mammography from a younger age.

A combination of regular self-breast examination and mammography provides the best screening for breast cancer. When an abnormality is picked up on mammography an ultrasound, which is a simple, non-invasive procedure, is sometimes recommended to determine whether the abnormality is solid or a cyst and provide further information. Discrete abnormalities are usually further investigated by needle aspiration. A fine needle is inserted into the localised abnormal region of the breast and a sample of cells removed. These are then examined by a pathologist.

Although a number of women are reluctant to undergo mammography for a variety of reasons, it cannot be emphasised enough that early detection is the key to breast cancer being a curable disease.

PREVENTING BREAST CANCER

Prevention of breast cancer involves modifying the behaviour and reproductive factors of a community of healthy women among whom individual risk cannot be precisely defined.

Simple plausible interventions to prevent breast cancer include:

- avoidance of breast radiation exposure, especially in adolescents;
- avoidance of passive and active cigarette smoking, particularly in adolescents;
- avoidance or minimal use of alcohol, particularly in younger women;

- long duration of lactation;
- nutritional modifications
  - having a high intake of vegetables, especially green leafy vegetables and cruciferous vegetables such as broccoli, cabbage and brussels sprouts;
  - incorporating soy products and other foods rich in phytoestrogens into the daily diet;
- exercise
  - avoiding obesity and participating in regular moderate exercise may modify oestrogen metabolism and decrease the likelihood of breast cancer.

It is more difficult at a community level to influence the length of the time between the start of menstruation and the age at which women have their first child. It has been estimated that a one year increase in the average age of menarche would result in a nine per cent decrease in the population-wide risk of breast cancer at the age of 70. Increased physical activity in prepubertal and adolescent girls is associated with later menarche and may be also related to a lower risk of premenopausal breast cancer. Avoidance of overeating and obesity in childhood and adolescence impacts on the timing of puberty and may reduce future breast cancer risk. Specific dietary components such as folate and vitamin A may protect the breast against cell damage during the interval of high cell turnover between menarche and the first full-term pregnancy. This is an important area of future research.

Recognition that the timing of the start of menstruation and adolescent exposure to toxins are perhaps the most important determinants of future breast cancer risk will hopefully lead to the refocusing of breast cancer prevention research. Young girls need to be taught about the importance of physical activity and the dangers of alcohol and smoking cigarettes.

DRUGS AND BREAST CANCER PREVENTION

The use of medications to prevent breast cancer is also being investigated. The drug tamoxifen, which is used in the treatment of breast cancer, is the focus of several prevention studies. Women at increased risk of breast cancer have been enrolled in these studies in order to determine whether taking tamoxifen will reduce the incidence of breast cancer over several years.

Non-steroidal, anti-inflammatory drugs (NSAIDs) like aspirin and ibuprofin may protect against the development of breast cancer. Women who have regularly used these medications at least three times a week for more than one year were observed to have a 34 per cent reduction in breast cancer risk compared with non-users. The greatest risk reduction was seen in women who took these drugs daily for more than five years. NSAIDs exert their effects by reducing the production of chemicals known as prostaglandins. Breast cancer cells produce prostaglandins, specifically prostaglandin E_2. This prostaglandin may, in turn, stimulate oestrogen production by breast fat cells. By blocking prostaglandin production in breast cancer cells, drugs like aspirin may turn off breast fat cell oestrogen production and ultimately limit breast cancer development or progression.

The most extreme method of preventing breast cancer in a woman at high risk is the complete surgical removal of both breasts. Despite the radical nature of this procedure, it is occasionally performed in women who are at very high risk of premenopausal breast cancer.

PREVENTIVE STRATEGIES

The ideal management approach to any disease process is prevention. Until recently the medical and scientific focus for breast cancer has been on diagnosis and treatment and prevention has been sadly underresearched. The dramatic differences in the incidences of breast cancer between various nations highlight the importance of environmental, reproductive, nutritional and lifestyle factors in the development of breast cancer. Priority must also be given to breast cancer prevention research, which now appears crucial to counteract the global increase in breast cancer in women.

8
HEART DISEASE

Cardiovascular disease is the main cause of death in women over the age of 50. In itself this is not surprising, as people must ultimately die, and in the older years stroke or coronary artery disease is the most common cause of death. But women in Westernised countries live longer on average than men, and as a consequence, they experience several more years of ill health and hence disability. More aggressive prevention and management of cardiovascular disease in women is likely to reduce the number of years spent suffering ill health and improve their quality of life. This chapter emphasises the following points.

- Coronary artery disease is *common* in women.
- Risk factors for cardiovascular disease and established coronary artery disease frequently go *undiagnosed* in women.
- Once diagnosed, women have a *higher* mortality from coronary artery disease than men.
- Women are *less* likely to receive aggressive therapy for an acute heart attack than men.
- Far *less* research has been conducted into cardiovascular disease in women than in men, and it has been inappropriately assumed that the knowledge regarding cardiovascular disease in men is applicable to women.
- There are risk factors and prevention strategies for cardiovascular disease, particularly coronary artery disease, that are *unique* to women.

In past years, the relationship between women and heart disease has normally been viewed in terms of women taking care of their husband's heart disease. Men are at greater risk of cardiovascular disease at a younger age. Women mostly develop significant coronary disease ten to fifteen years later than men, with a sharp increase in risk occurring after menopause. Beyond the age of 60 years the prevalence of coronary artery disease in women and men is equal.

Not uncommonly, the diagnosis of coronary artery disease is delayed in women. It has been suggested that this is because women experience different angina (heart) pain to men. This is not true. The classic pain of angina, caused by insufficient blood flowing to the heart muscle, is the same in both women and men. However, women often underrate and are dismissive of their symptoms, not considering that their pain could be attributable to a heart problem, and frequently underreport their symptoms to their doctor.

There is still a substantial gap in our knowledge of cardiovascular disease in women because of the limited number of studies published to date which have included women. Of those that have, the numbers of women involved have been mostly too few for clear conclusions to be drawn. Of the published studies addressing the benefits of lowering cholesterol in apparently healthy people, only 5800 of more than 30 000 participants have been women, and of the 43 main population studies designed to assess the relationship between exercise and coronary artery disease, only seven have included women. Despite differences between the sexes in the pattern of development of coronary artery disease, the medical and scientific communities have tended to automatically extrapolate the research findings on cardiovascular disease in men to women. Clearly, there can be major pitfalls in doing this. More research is urgently required to evaluate both cardiovascular risk factors and the effects of specific preventative practices such as aspirin therapy or anti-oxidant vitamins and different modes of treating established heart disease in women specifically.

The key to minimising cardiovascular disease is *prevention*. To gain the maximum benefit from preventative strategies it is necessary to understand what cardiovascular disease is, what causes it and who is at risk.

WHAT IS CARDIOVASCULAR DISEASE?

Cardiovascular disease is a term which encompasses disease of the arteries to the heart (the coronary arteries) and the other major arteries of the body, and in most instances develops as a result of *atherosclerosis*. Atherosclerosis is derived from the Greek words 'atheros' which means porridge and 'sclerosis' which means hardening. Thus atherosclerosis is hardening of the arteries as a result of porridge-like deposits. It is the build-up of fatty deposits in the lining of major arteries resulting in narrowing of these arteries and a lessening of the ability of the arteries to function normally, for example not dilating (opening up) when more blood flow is required during exercise. The term *generalised atherosclerosis* is often used, but this is misleading since different arteries are more affected at different stages of life. The aorta is usually affected earliest and most severely by atherosclerosis. The process of atherosclerosis is very gradual, developing over decades, with changes beginning in the aorta in early childhood. What are believed to be the first changes, known as *fatty streaks*, are present in all children, irrespective of race, gender or country of residence, by the age of 10. These early deposits of fat in the blood vessel lining may never progress, but if they do enlarge over the years, fatty deposits known as *atherosclerotic plaques*, the hallmark of atherosclerosis, develop. These are fibrous, firm, fat-filled 'lumps' in the lining of the arteries somewhat akin to a build-up of calcium salt in plumbing systems. Atherosclerosis not only limits blood flow by blockage but also by interfering with blood vessel function. Healthy arteries are able to constrict and dilate and do so to vary the flow of blood to different parts of the body according to need. During exercise the blood vessels supplying the heart muscle, the coronary arteries, dilate to increase the blood flow to match the demands of the hard working heart muscle. When there is significant atherosclerosis in the arteries, their function is impaired and they cannot dilate normally when the heart muscle demand increases during exercise. This results in chest pain with exercise known as angina. When an atherosclerotic deposit becomes sufficiently large it causes narrowing of the artery and limits blood flow through the artery even at rest. A heart attack (*myocardial infarction*) occurs when an artery to the heart muscle becomes critically narrowed or blocked and a region of the heart muscle dies. This is usually precipitated by rupture of a fatty deposit and sudden clotting of the blood in the blocked artery to the heart. Aspirin, which is an anti-clotting drug, is commonly prescribed to prevent this happening in high risk individuals. If a heart attack is detected early enough, special agents can be given in hospital intravenously to reverse the blood clotting process and dissolve the newly formed clot, thus limiting the extent of heart muscle damage. This is known as *thrombolysis* (clot breakdown) therapy. The same process of rupture of an atherosclerotic deposit and blood clotting can occur in one of the main arteries to the brain, resulting in a stroke, and, less commonly, in other major arteries of the body, leading to damage to the region supplied by the affected blood vessel. People at high risk for stroke are also usually prescribed daily aspirin as an anti-clotting agent as a preventive measure.

As already mentioned, all people develop fatty streaks in their arteries which only progress to frank atherosclerosis when there are other interacting factors. These include:

- untreated high blood pressure (hypertension);
- smoking tobacco;
- abnormal levels of cholesterol;
- elevated blood glucose (diabetes);

Over time all these factors cause injury to the arteries and their lining, which are also subject to unavoidable wear and tear with ageing. The other major irrevocable risk factor is having a strong family history of premature cardiovascular disease. Individuals with inherited risk need to be particularly attentive to limiting any other reversible risk conditions.

WHAT ABOUT THE RECENT DECLINE IN CARDIOVASCULAR DEATHS?

There has been a striking reduction in the rate of deaths from coronary heart disease in countries such as Australia and the US since the late 1960s. This trend partly reflects the success of public education campaigns aimed at heart disease prevention with focuses on dietary cholesterol and exercise. However, the greatest impact on the decline in deaths from coronary heart disease has been from advances in drug treatment and medical and surgical management of victims of heart disease. People suffering a first heart attack in the 1990s are far less likely to die as a result of their heart condition than people suffering equivalent ill health 30 years ago. Our understanding of the diseases and lifestyle factors which predispose the individual to cardiovascular disease such as high cholesterol, hypertension, diabetes and smoking, along with improved drug therapies, has resulted in more aggressive medical treatment of these conditions. Furthermore, the overall cholesterol levels of the adult populations of Australia and North America have fallen over the last few decades and fewer adult men are now smoking.

This is all good news, so should we still be concerned about cardiovascular disease? Things appear to be moving in the right direction with apparently reasonable community awareness and a declining mortality from coronary artery disease . . . *but*, it is naive to think this trend is certain to continue. The current reduction in cardiovascular deaths reflects the efficacy of health education and community life-style changes which occurred in the 1970s, combined with recent medical and technological advances. After the 1970s the population of the US started to become more overweight, although this change was gradual at first and its impact was therefore slight. From the mid-1980s there has been a sudden, dramatic increase in the body weight of the average North American with obesity becoming not only more common in adults but also in children and adolescents. Obesity is an established, major, predisposing condition for cardiovascular disease and adult-onset diabetes mellitus. Furthermore, while over this same time period there has been a decline in smoking of tobacco among men, this trend has not been observed among women who have continued to smoke. Young women, in particular, are smoking more and increasing their likelihood of developing coronary artery disease and lung cancer. Recent statistics confirm the danger of this trend in that lung cancer, not breast cancer, is now the leading cause of cancer death in American women.

So in terms of deaths attributable to heart disease, the benefits of the community health awareness and improved medical management of two decades ago are being observed now. The impact of public health issues such as obesity, increased rate of acquired diabetes and increased smoking in women will probably not be seen for a number of years. Countries like Australia and New Zealand usually lag behind the US by up to a decade in terms of population health trends and lifestyle patterns. In Australia we are only just beginning to see a major shift to high fat, calorie dense convenience food, increasingly sedentary existence and obesity, most worryingly in children and teenagers. Ten years ago, paediatricians were warning Australian parents of the dangers of having young children and adolescents on very low fat, 'Pritikin' style diets, but now things have swung completely the other way with frequent meals of McDonalds, KFC or other fast food becoming more the norm. The average weight of Australian twelve-year-old girls was three kilograms greater in 1994 than in 1985, while the average weight of fourteen-year-old boys increased six kilograms over the same period. Major factors causing this include declining physical activity and increased consumption of unhealthy food.

Consistent with this is the publication of recent research revealing an alarming *tenfold* increase in 'adult' type, non-insulin dependent diabetes mellitus in the teenage population of mid-west America over the last decade. The risk of developing diabetes doubles for every twenty per cent of excess body weight, and over 90 per cent of the teenagers who develop adult type diabetes are overweight, the vast majority being classifiable as obese. It is believed that it is this same combination of sedentary lifestyle and easy access to calorie dense food that results in teenage obesity and premature development of adult-type diabetes. It is feared that as this type of lifestyle is 'achieved' as predicted across the world, a similar increase in frequency in diabetes in adolescent populations in other countries will occur. Diabetes is a major cause of ill health, cardiovascular disease and premature death and the increasing frequency of the early onset of this disease will have significant future public health consequences.

The enthusiastic population trends of a decade ago towards health consciousness, good nutrition and exercise seem to have been swamped by the pressure of living. We can't afford to be complacent about the improvements we have observed in the medical statistics that show a reduction in deaths from cardiovascular disease. Instead we need to evaluate the *future* risks of heart disease for the community according to *current* lifestyle patterns, such as the increase in teenage and adult obesity and diabetes. Understanding the consequences of these conditions, as well as the significance of the other principal risk factors, is the first step towards preventing cardiovascular disease at both individual and community level.

RISK FACTORS FOR CARDIOVASCULAR DISEASE IN WOMEN AND MEN

Cardiovascular disease risk factors are usually classified as those that can be modified and those that cannot. Gender and family history, which obviously cannot be changed, are important. Having a strong family history of cardiovascular disease, that is having parents or siblings who have been affected, is a major risk factor, especially if the family member(s) have had disease at a young age (less than 60 years for women and less than 55 years for men).

The treatable risk factors for atherosclerosis and coronary artery disease in women and men include the following.

Major factors:

- cigarette smoking;
- hypertension;
- abnormal cholesterol parameters;
- diabetes mellitus;
- obesity (abdominal).

Minor factors:

- high triglycerides;
- sedentary lifestyle;
- high saturated fat intake;

The identified risk factors for stroke in women are:

- cigarette smoking;
- hypertension;
- high cholesterol.

Reversal of any of these important risk factors will significantly decrease the chance of a woman developing cardiovascular disease.

Cigarette smoking

Women who smoke twenty or more cigarettes per day are two to four times more likely to develop coronary heart disease than non-smokers. What is not commonly appreciated is that women who are light smokers, one to four cigarettes per day, also have double the risk of coronary heart disease than non-smokers. The good news is that when a person stops smoking completely, the risk of coronary heart disease begins to decrease within a few months and equals that of non-smokers after about five years irrespective of the number of cigarettes smoked per day or how long the individual has smoked. So it is never too late to give up.

Smoking is, unfortunately, very common among women, especially adolescents. There is a general belief that cigarettes with low tar and nicotine are less harmful, but in terms of heart disease risk, low-yield cigarettes are no safer than high-yield brands. Quite simply, women who smoke any form of tobacco, including tobacco mixed with marijuana, significantly increase their chance of developing cardiovascular disease.

Smokers also experience menopause on average one and a half years earlier than non-smokers, again irrespective of how heavily they smoke. Cigarette smoking affects body oestrogen metabolism, so that oestrogen is more likely to be converted to an inactive form in the body. Inactivation of oestrogen by nicotine also enhances bone loss and has a negative effect on blood vessels, and adds to the direct damaging effects of cigarette smoking on the arteries, heart and bones. In short, *any* form of cigarette smoking is bad news.

Hypertension

Elevated blood pressure increases the likelihood of stroke and coronary artery disease in both women and men and treatment of hypertension protects against both of these conditions. However, the side effects of blood pressure-lowering drugs have been less well studied in women than in men. There is a paucity of information about the control of blood pressure by non-pharmacological means such as diet, exercise and weight loss, specifically in women. Nevertheless, from the information available, which includes studies predominantly involving men, weight loss and exercise programs have been shown to lower blood pressure, as well as improve blood fat levels.

When blood pressure is measured, two values are recorded. The upper value is known as the *systolic* pressure and the lower value as the *diastolic* pressure. Doctors are mostly concerned when the diastolic blood pressure is raised and it is well established that chronically elevated diastolic blood pressure should be treated. There is a tendency for physicians to be dismissive of elevated systolic pressure, which is called *systolic hypertension*. It is due to loss of elasticity of the arteries and is clearly associated with increased risk of death from stroke and coronary heart disease. This condition is more common in women and frequently goes untreated. Systolic hypertension in women should be treated in order to reduce the possibility of stroke and coronary heart disease.

Blood pressure problems commonly first develop in women during pregnancy, and it is vital that all women who experience elevated blood pressure in pregnancy have a formal, follow-up medical examination, appropriate investigations performed and treatment instituted if high blood pressure persists for some time after delivery. Many young women seem to end up taking blood pressure medication without ever being fully investigated. This is not good practice as occasionally underlying correctable causes of elevated blood pressure are detected by specific tests.

Cholesterol in women

Cholesterol is a compound found only in animals, not in plants, which plays a vital role in the structure of all normal animal cells. It also circulates in the blood bound to special proteins. High levels of circulating cholesterol in humans are unequivocally associated with the development of cardiovascular disease. Cholesterol is either absorbed in the diet from animal products or produced by the liver. High blood cholesterol levels usually develop not because people eat too much cholesterol but because they eat too much *saturated fat*. The body can deal with dietary cholesterol, within reason, but saturated (animal) fat is converted by the liver into blood cholesterol. Saturated fats are found in meat fats, dairy fats, biscuits, cakes and especially in convenience and take-away foods. Some people can cope better with excessive dietary fat than others because the rate at which the liver converts fat into cholesterol is highly genetically determined. However, the type of food consumed is a major influence on cholesterol levels in all people.

Blood 'lipids' is a term which includes total cholesterol, various subgroups of cholesterol and other blood fats. Although too much fat is a bad thing, cholesterol and fat are important components of human nutrition. Cholesterol is important for cell growth and stability and blood fats are needed for the absorption of the fat soluble vitamins A, D and E, as well as for the storage and transport of energy.

The metabolism of blood fats and cholesterol is complex and dynamic. Many subtypes of cholesterol and fat circulate in the blood, but the ones most routinely measured are *total cholesterol* and *triglycerides*. It is not necessary to be fasting to measure blood cholesterol; however, triglyceride levels fluctuate significantly after food, therefore an accurate triglyceride value requires a blood sample after an overnight fast. Triglycerides are the fats in food which are classified as being 'saturated', 'monounsaturated' or 'polyunsaturated'. Unlike cholesterol, the role of triglycerides, and the impact of high levels of triglycerides on the development of cardiovascular disease, are still controversial.

The main measured components of total cholesterol are *low density* (LDL) and *high density* (HDL) cholesterol. LDL-cholesterol is often described as the harmful form of cholesterol. High LDL-cholesterol increases the risk of atherosclerosis, and this risk is even greater in people with a high proportion of small, dense LDL-cholesterol molecules. *Oxidised* forms of LDL-cholesterol are also particularly harmful. Oxidised LDL directly irritates and injures the lining of blood vessels and is more likely to be deposited in the blood vessel wall.

HDL-cholesterol is often called the good form of cholesterol. It acts as a system for removing cholesterol from the tissues and transporting it back to the liver and therefore high levels of HDL-cholesterol are associated with reduced risk of cardiovascular disease. HDL-cholesterol is one of the most *significant* markers of risk for cardiovascular disease in women. Low HDL-cholesterol levels are associated with a several-fold increase in the risk of a woman developing coronary artery disease.

When total cholesterol is found to be elevated (greater than 5.5 mmol/l) further measurements should be made to determine whether this is due to increased HDL or LDL-cholesterol. Often HDL-cholesterol is found to be raised and LDL-cholesterol is normal. If this is the case, the patient can be reassured. If the problem is high LDL-cholesterol, then it is appropriate to try to lower this level. Ideally, this should be accomplished by modifying eating habits, exercise and weight reduction. Occasionally, special cholesterol-lowering medication is required.

There is increasing evidence that aggressive treatment of elevated LDL-cholesterol in people with clear-cut cardio-vascular disease can actually result in reversal of the disease process and regression of fatty deposits in arteries. Possibly more importantly, lowering cholesterol in individuals with high cholesterol levels improves blood vessel function, and this is vital in terms of preventing angina and heart attacks.

The controversy regarding the significance of elevated cholesterol in women prevails, and there is a tendency for high cholesterol in women to be undertreated. The problem resides in the paucity of published data on cholesterol in women. The Scandinavian Simvastatin Survival Study, also known as the 4S Study, is considered to be the landmark study which demonstrated that reducing cholesterol in people with known coronary artery disease will reduce deaths, but only nineteen per cent of those involved were women. Although this study showed a reduction in overall deaths in those treated with cholesterol-lowering medication, this did not hold for the women. The *female* death rate in this study was *no* different between those treated with cholesterol-lowering and those not treated (the control or placebo group). Further studies of numbers of women are needed to prove that treatment of women with coronary artery disease and high cholesterol will increase life expectancy.

We know even less about the value of treating women with high cholesterol who have no known coronary artery disease. There is no published medical data which addresses this issue. We do know that in women without heart disease *low* HDL-cholesterol is a much stronger risk factor for the development of heart disease than *high* LDL-cholesterol. This may be a fundamental difference between men and women.

In contrast to the incomplete evidence supporting the use of cholesterol-lowering drugs in women, there are numerous published studies indicating a 30 to 50 per cent reduction in mortality from coronary artery disease in post-menopausal women who use oestrogen replacement (see pages 191–5). Continuous oestrogen replacement taken orally, even in combination with progesterone taken continuously, significantly lowers total and LDL-cholesterol and increases HDL-cholesterol (in post-menopausal women with high cholesterol). These effects are comparable to those seen with cholesterol-lowering drugs. In addition, HRT significantly reduces a form of cholesterol called *lipoprotein (a)* which is strongly linked with cardiovascular disease but unaffected by most other cholesterol-lowering therapies. Therefore post-menopausal women with elevated blood cholesterol levels should consider hormone replacement therapy ahead of other cholesterol-lowering medications.

Is low cholesterol dangerous?

Very low cholesterol levels are seen in some forms of cancer, lung and liver disease. In contrast, some healthy individuals have 'naturally occurring' low cholesterol throughout life. People with lifelong, low cholesterol are not at increased risk of cancer and other diseases. However, people who have middle-range or high levels of cholesterol throughout life may have a dramatic reduction in their cholesterol when they develop cancer or liver disease. The low cholesterol is not a cause of the disease but an effect of the ill health. It appears that a drop in serum cholesterol sometimes occurs over a decade before the disease, for example cancer, is diagnosed.

Cholesterol and diet

In the past we have been told to eat less fat in order to lower cholesterol. We are now more aware that the *type* of fat is probably more important than the *quantity*. Australians eat a very high proportion of *saturated* fat, mainly from palm oil and tallow (beef fat). Unlike saturated fats which increase blood cholesterol, *unsaturated* fats like canola oil, sunflower oil and olive oil have been found to have a cholesterol-lowering effect and may even be 'protective' against heart disease. For example, Mediterranean communities which traditionally consume considerable amounts of olive oil have a low rate of heart disease. This does not mean that such fats should be consumed indiscriminately, but that they are a more suitable form to use in food preparation.

Another class of fats which are receiving a lot of attention are *trans fats*. These are artificial fats used in a variety of manufactured and take-away foods. They have no nutritional qualities, but when consumed regularly cause LDL-cholesterol to increase and HDL-cholesterol to fall, and they have been linked to the development of coronary artery disease. If possible, trans fats should be avoided, and it is wise to look at labels of commercial products, especially margarines, to check that they are free of trans fats. Beware the 'cholesterol free' claim of many prepackaged or convenience foods. These foods may contain little or no cholesterol but still be high in saturated fat, which the body will then convert into cholesterol. Low cholesterol does not mean a product is low in calories or low in fat. Also, be aware that 'low' fat foods are not always fat free. Furthermore, in order to make low fat products palatable, gums, water, artificial flavours and preservatives are usually added, and we do not know the long-term health effects of eating these unnatural products.

Soon *olestra*, or fake fat, will be available for use. This is a synthetic 'fat-free' fat which has now been approved as a food additive in the US. Olestra appears to affect the availability of the fat soluble vitamins A and E, which are believed to be important anti-cancer vitamins. Widespread use of olestra in convenience and snack food could be very dangerous in the long term. As already stated, nothing can replace the nutritional value of natural fresh grains, fruits and vegetables, which are the only truly safe forms of low fat, low cholesterol and low calorie food.

Diabetes mellitus

Diabetes is a major risk factor for coronary artery disease in women; in fact, it is an even *stronger* risk factor for women than men. Diabetes in the premenopausal years even overrides the protective effects of oestrogen against cardiovascular disease. Diabetes also enhances the other risk factors for cardiovascular disease such as hypertension, smoking and obesity and reversal of these risk factors is of even greater benefit to diabetics than to the rest of the population. Women who have transient diabetes during pregnancy are more likely to develop high blood pressure, elevated blood fats and diabetes later in life, and need to pay particular attention to the prevention of these conditions.

Total body weight and cardiovascular risk

Until recently, obesity has been considered a minor risk factor for cardiovascular disease but this view represents an under-estimation of the impact of body weight on atherosclerosis. Being severely obese is clearly a cause of ill health, but the health consequences of being moderately overweight to mildly obese have been the subject of intense debate. When considering the health risks of varying body weights we must take into account *total body weight* with an adjustment for *height* and where the fat is deposited in the body, which is known as *body fat distribution*.

Total body weight is adjusted for individual height by a simple formula resulting in a calculated value called the *body mass index* or BMI. Using BMI rather than total body weight enables more realistic comparison of weight or fatness between individuals. BMI equals total weight measured in kilograms divided by height measured in metres, squared (kg/m²). A normal BMI for a Caucasian is 20 to 25 kg/m². A value of 26 to 30 kg/m² is considered overweight and above 30 kg/m² obese.

Having a high BMI is a health hazard. Women who have a BMI of 32 kg/m² or more who have never smoked have four times the risk of death from cardiovascular disease and double the risk of cancer than women with a BMI of 19 kg/m². Put in perspective, being obese is at least as significant a risk factor for cardiovascular disease as smoking twenty or more cigarettes per day. Weight gain during adulthood is also detrimental, and the belief that it is normal to gain weight with increasing age is a myth which must be dispelled. Women who gain ten kilograms or more after the age of eighteen are at increased risk of death from all causes during their middle years. Also contrary to popular belief, leanness is not associated with increased mortality. In fact, women who are lean, that is weigh at least fifteen per cent less than the average North American woman and whose weight has been stable since early adulthood, have the *lowest* death rate. Low body weight is the only factor consistently linked to longevity in all populations studied.

Body fat distribution

Where excessive fat is stored is far more important than the total amount of fat a person has. Excessive weight is associated with diabetes, high blood pressure, elevated blood cholesterol and triglycerides and atherosclerosis, but not all overweight individuals develop these conditions.

During their reproductive years women tend to store their fat around their bottoms and thighs, hence the healthy, feminine pear-shape most women these days detest. This fat is metabolically 'inactive', and having an increased quantity of *lower-body* fat does not result in elevated cholesterol and is not linked to atherosclerosis. The storage of fat in the lower body in women is probably under the influence of oestrogen, and appears to confer an evolutionary, biological, survival advantage. This 'healthy' fat store in times past would have been an important potential energy source for women to see them through pregnancy, breastfeeding and childcaring during times of famine or illness.

Men, in contrast, have little bottom or thigh fat and store their excessive fat around the waist and upper body. Fat stored in these regions is highly metabolically 'active', especially the fat stores deep in the abdomen known as *deep* or *visceral* fat.

- The more deep abdominal fat a person has, the greater their likelihood of having raised blood cholesterol and triglycerides, elevated blood insulin and therefore of developing atherosclerosis and diabetes. The different way in which men and women in their reproductive years store fat is a major factor in the gender differences in circulating blood fats (cholesterol and triglycerides) and development of atherosclerosis between women and men. Premenopausal women can accumulate more total body fat than men of the same age without achieving an equivalent amount of deep abdominal fat because it nearly all goes to their hips.

In urbanised societies people tend to gain weight as they grow older. Whether this is part of the natural ageing process or due to a more sedentary lifestyle with increasing age is not clear. Information from hunter–gather societies suggests that weight gain with age is not natural for humans but due to lifestyle. Natural menopause is associated with loss of fat-free body weight (for example, muscle mass) and an increase in total body fat. Theoretically these should balance out and total weight shouldn't change. However, one study has shown that after menopause women are less likely to be physically active during leisure time compared with women of the same age who have not experienced menopause. Not surprisingly, the greatest weight gain occurs in women who have the most marked decline in exercise. We do not know why this observed lifestyle change occurs. As women gain weight after meno-pause, the fat is no longer laid down around the hips and bottom as there is insufficient oestrogen circulating to direct it to the hips. Therefore post-menopausal women are more likely to accumulate unhealthy abdominal fat.

Stored abdominal fat is somewhat 'resistant' to the actions of insulin. The more abdominal fat, the greater the insulin resistance and then the body has to make excessive insulin to cope with this resistance. Insulin resistance associated with excessive abdominal fat is linked to elevated LDL-cholesterol and triglycerides and low HDL-cholesterol and is a strong predisposing factor for atherosclerosis and cardiovascular dis-ease.

High levels of insulin in women with abdominal obesity during the reproductive years can also cause disturbances of ovulation. This is because excess insulin stimulates the cells of the ovaries to overproduce androgens (testosterone), which interferes with ovulation. Menstruation becomes irregular and a condition of polycystic ovaries with excessive body hair and infertility may result (see Chapter 4).

It is often said that post-menopausal hormone replace-ment therapy leads to weight gain. There is absolutely no evidence to support this. Urbanised women tend to gain weight around mid-life irrespective of HRT use. The oestro-gen of HRT may favour fat deposition in the lower body, which as we know is healthier, but a feature about which many women complain.

The degree of abdominal obesity is often determined by the ratio between waist and hip circumference; however, waist circumference alone is an excellent indication of the amount of fat stored in the abdomen. The complications of obesity, namely hypertension, diabetes and high blood lipids, are more likely when waist circumference exceeds 100 cm.

People who suffer abdominal and upper body weight excess can markedly improve their health by modifying what they eat by restricting calories, and undertaking exercise.

Dietary restriction and weight loss will result in a preferential loss of abdominal fat, thereby reducing cardiovascular risk. In terms of exercise, the standard exercise program that used to be recommended to improve cardio-respiratory fitness was three sessions of 20 minutes endurance exercise per week, but vigorous exercise is not necessary and this short duration will not generate enough energy expenditure to have a significant effect on body fatness. Modification of total body fatness and reduction of abdominal fat requires low intensity, prolonged exercise of at least 45 minutes per session on a nearly daily basis (according to recent recommendation by the American College of Sports Medicine and the Centers for Disease Control and Prevention, USA). The *duration* and the *regularity* of the exercise are most important.

For women, the oestrogen lack after menopause is inevitable and this adversely affects body fat distribution, blood cholesterol levels, insulin action and, as an end point, the risk of cardiovascular disease. Although oestrogen replacement can to some extent combat these changes it is no substitute for attention to the food eaten or regular exercise for the prevention of inappropriate weight gain and accumulation of abdominal fat with increasing age.

EVOLUTION AND THE ENVIRONMENT—AN EXTREME EXAMPLE OF THE DANGERS OF WESTERNISED LIFESTYLE

No community has been as dramatically affected by Westernisation as the Australian Aboriginal people who have been literally catapulted into the late twentieth century from their traditional lifestyle as hunter–gatherers. As such Aboriginal Australians were extremely physically fit and lean (body mass index less than 20 kg/m^2) and, consistent with the physical demands of their lifestyle, their weight did not increase with age. They had low blood glucose and low cholesterol, as well as low blood pressure, and apparently no diabetes or cardio-vascular disease. Even though traditionally living Aboriginal people are lean (often with BMIs of 14 to 17 kg/m^2, whereas a normal Caucasian BMI is said to be 20 to 25 kg/m^2) they are not malnourished but generally very healthy. In contrast, most Australian Aboriginal people today lead sedentary lives, eat mostly calorie dense, Western style food, are commonly obese and are often malnourished. The prevalence of diabetes and heart disease among Aborigines is ten-fold and four-fold that of the rest of the Australian population respectively and they have a life expectancy twenty years shorter than other Australians. Fundamentally, radical lifestyle changes have resulted in previously unknown diseases becoming common-place among these people. Premenopausal Aboriginal women tend to accumulate abdominal fat when they gain weight, in contrast to Caucasian women who are more likely to gain fat around their hips and thighs, which explains their suscepti-bility to the health problems arising from obesity. In order to maintain good health Aboriginal women need to maintain a lower body weight than their non-Aboriginal Australian counterparts.

In terms of disease prevention, we should learn a great deal from the effects that physical inactivity and obesity have had on Aboriginal health. The stark reality is that what has happened to Aboriginal people in only a few years has been happening more gradually to people of European descent over the last century, and which has now almost become culturally acceptable. Traditionally fit Aboriginal people were obviously unaware that the dietary restrictions and low intensity, pro-longed exercise which were integral parts of their lives were protecting them from cardiovascular disease. This 'formula' for disease prevention is no different from that recommended for non-Aboriginal people with problems of abdominal obesity.

In most Asian populations BMI is also low (often less than 20 kg/m^2 as seen in healthy Aborigines), although a trend of increasing BMI with increasing Westernisation and affluence is being observed. This tendency towards greater weight in Asian countries among individuals with higher socio-economic status is also associated with higher blood pressure and blood cholesterol levels. Preventing future increases in average weight in populations where average body weight is still low may be fundamental for preventing major, large-scale adverse health consequences, such as cardiovascular disease and diabetes, in the next decades.

It is important to understand that not long ago in terms of evolution we were all hunters and gatherers and, despite some ethnic differences, like the Aboriginal people we are not naturally physically adapted to our Western lifestyle, which is unhealthy for each one of us. People who restrict their food intake, within reason, and exercise regularly are not food faddists and 'health freaks' but are reproducing for themselves the important components of the ancient hunter–gatherer lifestyle to which the human body is still ideally suited.

Physical activity

Consistent with this and reinforcing what has been stated elsewhere, *prolonged* physical activity in women has been found to be more cardiovascularly beneficial than the usually recommended 20 to 30 minutes of moderate regular exercise. In terms of jogging, the further athletic women run per week the higher their HDL-cholesterol and the lower their waist size, two major predictors of protection from heart disease in women. High intensity exercise is not necessary to achieve improvements in blood cholesterol levels, rather the frequency of exercise appears to be far more important. Older people take longer to achieve the benefits of exercise than younger individuals. Improvements in HDL-cholesterol levels may not be seen for as much as two years after regular exercise is begun by people over the age of 50 years, compared to effects seen after six to twelve months of regular exercise in younger women and men. Regular, prolonged (greater than 40 minutes) brisk walking is something virtually everyone can achieve.

As repeatedly emphasised, the information can be presented, but it is up to each woman to decide her priorities and the extent to which she chooses to be in control of her health. Most people *can* exercise and should, but not everyone chooses to do so. As for all things, the greater the investment (in exercise) the greater the reward.

HORMONES AND THE CARDIOVASCULAR SYSTEM IN WOMEN

It's somewhat sobering to note that the first study of oestrogen replacement as a therapeutic approach for the prevention of coronary artery disease and heart attacks involved only *male* subjects. This reflects a focus on cardiovascular disease in men, as opposed to women, which dominated research in heart disease for many decades. This study of oestrogen replacement in men with previous heart attacks, which was published in the *Journal of the American Medical Association* in 1970, was prematurely aborted because of the higher rate of non-fatal adverse effects among oestrogen treated men. The oestrogen used was of a much higher dose than that recommended for hormone replacement therapy in women. The results of this study are not conclusive and, in any case, are not applicable to women.

As already discussed, women tend to develop cardiovascular disease later in life than men, and at a slower rate. The observation some years ago that surgical menopause (removal of both ovaries) and the accompanying dramatic lowering of blood oestrogen levels doubles the risk of coronary artery disease, and that oestrogen replacement removes this increased risk, implied a relationship between oestrogen and cardiovascular disease in women. Natural menopause appears to be linked with an increase in cardiovascular disease,

although this has not been statistically proven. Natural menopause is associated with a very gradual decline in oestrogen
levels over several years, and therefore any distinct relationship between reduced oestrogen levels and heart disease is
diluted over time and merges with the effects of ageing.
Consequently, it is difficult to clearly make an association
between the oestrogen loss with natural menopause and
cardiovascular disease which is separate from the effects of
ageing.

There is now a strong body of evidence which shows that
normal reproductive levels of oestrogen are needed for normal
cardiovascular function in women, and that oestrogen lack
may be a factor in the development of cardiovascular disease.
Variations in oestrogen levels during normal menstrual cycles
appear to affect parameters of cardiovascular function of
regularly ovulating women. This indicates the effects of oestrogen in women are not simply all or none but are extremely
complex, with subtle effects resulting from variations in
oestrogen levels within the normal range for young healthy
women.

Many published epidemiological studies consistently
demonstrate that post-menopausal oestrogen replacement
reduces the risk of cardiovascular disease by 30 to 50 per
cent. This protective effect is seen in fit, healthy women with
no risk factors. However, women who have the greatest risk
for cardiovascular disease appear to have the greatest benefit
from oestrogen therapy. Still, it should be noted that these
studies involved women who chose themselves whether or not
to use HRT. The women who used oestrogen were mostly
healthier and probably at lower risk of cardiovascular disease,
and thus the true protective effect of oestrogen in post-menopausal women may be somewhat less than what is suggested
by these studies.

There are several factors which contribute to the increased
rate of cardiovascular disease after menopause. These include:

- increases in body weight;
- redistribution of body fat so there is a tendency to more abdominal fat;
- changes in blood fats with increases in total cholesterol, LDL-cholesterol and triglycerides, and a fall in HDL-cholesterol;
- adverse changes in insulin metabolism which are linked to redistribution of body fat and change in body weight;
- loss of the direct beneficial effects that oestrogen has on blood vessels and cardiac function.

It is believed that oestrogen may protect women against the development of cardiovascular disease by various different mechanisms. Post-menopausal oestrogen use partially reverses some of the adverse changes in cholesterol and other blood fats that occur with oestrogen insufficiency. Total and LDL-cholesterol fall, HDL-cholesterol increases and a number of other positive metabolic effects of oestrogen on blood fat metabolism are observed. Oestrogen taken in tablet form may cause triglyceride levels to increase, although this is not usually a problem except for women who already have high triglyceride levels. Progestogens to some degree reverse this triglyceride effect. When oestrogen is taken by patch (transdermal) or implant, blood triglycerides do not change.

Only approximately one-third of the reduction in risk of coronary heart disease appears to be due to the modification of blood fats by oestrogen, however. There are several other important ways by which oestrogen may exert its protective effects.

- Oestrogen has been observed to have direct, positive effects on the function of the cells lining the arteries. This favours increased blood flow, as well as a reduction in the build-up of cholesterol deposits in the artery wall.
- Oestrogen may act as anti-oxidant, decreasing the formation of harmful, oxidised LDL-cholesterol and ultimately resulting in less atherosclerosis.

- Oestrogen may prevent thrombosis (blood clotting) in the coronary arteries of the heart.
- Oestrogen has been observed in some studies to have direct favourable action on the heart resulting in more effective heart muscle function and blood flow to the body.

There is no evidence that oestrogen replacement therapy causes weight gain. As we have already seen, women tend to gain weight in their middle years irrespective of whether or not they take HRT. Post-menopausal oestrogen may improve glucose and carbohydrate metabolism and reduce abdominal fat deposition, although this is still controversial and requires further study.

There have been concerns that progestogens, which are needed to be taken with oestrogen to protect the uterus from overstimulation and the risk of uterine cancer, may negate some of the beneficial effects of oestrogen. In fact, progestogens oppose the increase in blood triglycerides caused by oral oestrogen therapy and this is beneficial. Progestogens do not appear to negate the favourable effects of oestrogen of preventing cholesterol accumulation in arteries. Whether progestogens have any direct adverse effects on blood vessels remains unclear.

HORMONES AND WOMEN WITH HEART DISEASE

In the past, women who have had coronary artery disease have been told never to take oestrogen. We now know that such women appear to gain the greatest cardiovascular benefits from oestrogen replacement. The major studies of post-menopausal women with known coronary artery disease have shown greatly improved life expectancy in those who take oestrogen compared with those who do not. Again, these results must be viewed with some reservations as it is not clear what factors determine why women in these studies chose to take oestrogen or whether the women most at risk were advised against HRT.

It is important to note that oestrogen starts to protect against cardiovascular disease very soon after it is commenced and current users (as opposed to past users) have the maximum benefit. The immediate effects of oestrogen are probably related to its direct action on the blood vessels and their function. Therefore women do not need to start oestrogen at menopause in order to achieve the cardiovascular benefits. Starting HRT several years after menopause will still result in improved cardiovascular function, and this appears to be an important treatment option for all post-menopausal women with high cardiovascular risk or established disease.

There are several important recommendations regarding HRT and cardiovascular disease in menopausal and post-menopausal women.

- For women at low risk of cardiovascular disease, prevention of cardiovascular disease alone is not sufficient reason to use HRT long-term.
- All women who experience premature menopause (before the age of 40) should be on oestrogen to prevent their otherwise very high risk of premature atherosclerosis and cardiovascular disease. Women with an early menopause (between 40 and 45) are also often advised to take oestrogen for the same reasons.
- For treatment of high cholesterol, HRT should be considered before other cholesterol-lowering medications for post-menopausal women with or without known cardiovascular disease.
- For women at high risk or with known cardiovascular disease, HRT should be considered, particularly by women with angina or past heart attacks.

It is too simplistic to assume that when oestrogen is taken by women as HRT it is just 'replacing' what the ovaries no longer adequately produce. No medicine can be a true substitute for the natural production of oestrogen by the female ovary. Research clearly supports an important role for oestrogen produced by the ovaries in female cardiovascular health. However, it must be recognised that part of the beneficial action of oestrogen when taken as HRT may be pharmacological. For example, *conjugated equine oestrogen* (Premarin) contains a mixture of oestrogens, some of which appear to be more potent than naturally produced human ovarian oestrogen on blood cholesterol metabolism in women. Thus, it may be more accurate to talk about oestrogen therapy instead of oestrogen replacement therapy. This concept does not detract from the health benefits of oestrogen therapy but acknowledges that it is a medical treatment.

WHY IS CARDIOVASCULAR DISEASE MORE LETHAL IN WOMEN THAN MEN?

Once diagnosed, heart disease appears to be more lethal in women than in men. American statistics reveal that one year following hospital admission for heart disease, one-third of women have died but only one-quarter of men have died. Is this because the disease affects the sexes differently or is their treatment different?

Women do differ from men by having a later onset of coronary disease, therefore those admitted to hospital are likely to be older and hence have a higher subsequent mortality. Some American research suggests that there is differential treatment of men and women admitted to hospital after an acute heart attack, even in the 1990s. There is no evidence to suggest that this is a result of conscious gender bias. Thrombolytic (blood clot dissolving) treatment is still more likely to be given to male than female patients according to a report from the Minnesota Heart Survey Registry (American Heart Association Conference on Cardiovascular Disease, Epidemiology and Prevention, 1996). Overall, men were observed to be 43 per cent more likely than women to receive this form of therapy, which limits the extent of heart muscle damage. It is not clear what determines this differential management. Women also have a higher mortality when it comes to coronary artery surgery. Major factors for this are the greater age of women coming to surgery and that women have smaller arteries which are frequently extensively diseased, thus making surgery more technically difficult. Similar sex differences in survival are seen in women with the procedure of *coronary angioplasty*, in which a balloon is fed into the diseased coronary artery using a guide wire that is introduced into the body in the groin. The in-hospital death rate of women having this procedure is 50 per cent higher than for men; however, once discharged from hospital, the long-term success of this procedure for women is equal to that of men.

In summary, because women suffer heart disease later in life than men and because they are smaller than men and have smaller blood vessels, they are more likely to die from their disease. However, differential treatment of women with cardiovascular disease persists, and it is essential that discriminatory health care not only be recognised but eradicated.

NUTRITIONAL SUPPLEMENTS AND CARDIOVASCULAR DISEASE

Conventional belief has been that vitamin and mineral supplementation will not improve health if people have a balanced diet. However, there is now substantial evidence that anti-oxidants taken as supplements protect against cardiovascular disease, as well as against various cancers. Anti-oxidant vitamins include the fat soluble carotenoids (provitamin A), the vitamin E family (tocopherols and tocotrienols) and vitamin C. Other antioxidants occur ubiquitously in foods, particularly vegetables, and are now the focus of much research.

The anti-oxidant actions of all these compounds is extremely complex and the interaction between different anti-oxidants appears to be important for optimal effects to be achieved, for example vitamins E and C act in a complementary manner. Anti-oxidants consumed as food rather than as supplements are probably more likely to achieve the desired effect. This has been seen in breast cancer research in which low breast cancer risk was observed among women who had a high food intake of anti-oxidant vitamins but not among those who had the same vitamin intake in the form of supplements.

A high intake of vitamin E has been associated with a lower risk of coronary artery disease in women and men. However, a higher intake of vitamin E is also associated with an overall healthier lifestyle and lower heart disease risk; for example, by consuming more polyunsaturated fat and less saturated animal fat. These widely publicised studies have resulted in an enormous number of people now regularly taking vitamin E, but this practice is not backed by proof, only limited circumstantial evidence which warrants further investigation. Of concern is an increased risk of haemorrhagic stroke (a bleed into the brain tissue) among men taking vitamin E supplements observed in a Finnish Cancer Prevention study. It is not known whether the findings of this study are also applicable to women. High dose vitamin E is known to exacerbate high blood pressure, and vitamin E supplements should only be taken in low dose and under medical supervision by people with elevated blood pressure, diabetes or heart conditions.

The relationship between vitamin C supplements and cardiovascular disease prevention is even more controversial. Large population studies have not found vitamin C to be protective, whereas smaller studies provide limited support for the hypothesis that dietary vitamin C may protect against atherosclerosis.

Before widespread long-term use of vitamin supplements can be safely recommended the potential hazards of such therapies must be fully known. There is no information showing that the long-term intake of large doses of 'natural' anti-oxidants is safe. Therefore, despite the prevailing public and scientific enthusiasm for the potential cardiovascular benefits of anti-oxidant supplements, data to support this is incomplete and the possibility remains that the potential adverse effects have been underestimated.

Does fish contribute to heart disease prevention?

The low death rate from cardiovascular disease among the Inuit of Greenland and inhabitants of Okinawa in Japan, two communities with high fish consumption, generated the initial interest in the role of fish in coronary heart disease prevention. fish, particularly deep sea, oily fish and marine animals such as seals, are rich in a special type of polyunsaturated fat called omega-3 fatty acids. Initially, it was found that omega-3 fats lowered blood triglyceride levels and reduced blood clotting. Several other studies found that individuals who regularly consumed fish in other countries, namely Holland and the USA, had a low rate of coronary heart disease, the benefits being seen with as little as one to two fish meals per week. One of the mechanisms by which fish oil appears to exert its protective effect is by increasing the capacity of the cells lining blood vessels to produce factors (such as nitric oxide) which cause the blood vessels to dilate, and thereby enable the blood to flow more freely. In summary, evidence to date supports the idea that regular fish consumption is protective against cardiovascular disease and should be encouraged. A daily intake of fish may be no more effective than two meals per week, and fish oil supplements should be reserved for people being treated by their physicians for specific abnormalities of blood fats.

STROKE IN WOMEN

Stroke occurs when one of the main arteries supplying the brain is blocked or blood pressure builds up and a blood vessel bursts and bleeds. Thus the two main forms of stroke are *ischaemic* stroke (insufficient blood and therefore oxygen reaching the brain) due to a blocked artery, or *haemorrhagic* stroke (bleed into the brain). The major predisposing conditions for stroke in women and men are:

- high blood pressure;
- elevated cholesterol;
- smoking;
- strong family history of stroke.

Stroke is more common in women than in men and after the age of 65 is the cause of death for one-quarter of women. Controlling blood pressure and treating systolic hypertension are essential for the prevention of stroke.

Being at high risk for stroke was previously believed to be a contraindication to hormone replacement therapy; however, the reverse now appears to apply. *Oestrogen therapy* increases blood flow to the *carotid* arteries to the brain as well as reducing cholesterol build-up in these arteries. Oestrogen replacement in post-menopausal women at high risk has been observed to be associated with less frequent stroke and death due to stroke in some studies. To date most of the available knowledge is of women taking oestrogen alone and it is yet unclear whether or not the addition of progesterone interferes with the possible beneficial effects of oestrogen. Preliminary evidence shows the same reduction in risk of stroke for women taking combined oestrogen and progestogen therapy as seen in women taking oestrogen alone. However, more information regarding the effects of HRT on stroke is still needed before clear recommendations can be made.

Low dose aspirin, prescribed as an anti-clotting agent, reduces the incidence of heart attack, stroke and death from cardiovascular disease in both women and men who have had previous cardiovascular episodes. Studies in men have shown that men at high risk of coronary artery disease are less likely to have a heart attack if they take aspirin, but *no equivalent study has been done in women*. Many women are being prescribed aspirin as a preventative measure against heart attack and stroke with no solid basis for this practice. Clarification of the appropriate use of aspirin in women is essential as the risks of long-term aspirin may outweigh the benefits, in contrast to men. For example, although aspirin may reduce the risk of heart attack it may increase the risk of haemorrhagic stroke in women.

HEART DISEASE: THE FACTS

Cardiovascular disease is not the same in women and men:

- the clinical patterns of disease differ;
- the risk factors vary;
- the effect of the hormonal changes with menopause impact on the development of cardiovascular disease in women;
- the risks of surgical intervention are greater in women;
- the benefits of different treatment strategies differ between women and men;
- there are prevention and management options, such as the use of HRT, which are unique to women.

Without doubt, ceasing cigarette smoking, maintaining a normal body weight and avoiding excessive abdominal fat, being physically active and controlling blood pressure will minimise the likelihood of women developing cardiovascular disease. Furthermore:

- HDL cholesterol appears to be the best predictor of coronary heart disease in women, with low levels being linked to increased risk.
- A large body of evidence in men has shown that cholesterol reduction reduces mortality from coronary artery disease, and it is highly likely that this applies equally to women. However, there has not yet been a study published that absolutely shows this benefit for women.
- Oestrogen replacement after the menopause has beneficial effects on blood cholesterol and appears to reduce the death rate from coronary artery disease.
- The benefits for women of low dose aspirin, small amounts of alcohol and anti-oxidant vitamins in preventing coronary artery disease are not clearly established and more research is needed to evaluate the roles of these approaches.

The challenge for each woman is to achieve a healthy lifestyle and to avoid or change the elements which put her at risk for cardiovascular disease. It is also not only the responsibility of each of us to attend to these important aspects of our own health, but to pass on the knowledge and practice of good health to our sons and daughters.

SEXUALITY, ANDROGENS AND ANDROGEN THERAPY

In Westernised cultures which extol youthfulness, sexuality is perceived as a facet of life restricted to people up to their middle years, and it is rarely associated with older people whose sexuality is often invisible. Nevertheless, sexuality is an integral part of the human psyche and is present from birth to the grave, in all people.

It is essential therefore to acknowledge that human sexuality is much more than hormones, intercourse, procreation and orgasm. Sexuality is expressed throughout life in all people, both consciously and unconsciously, in body movements, body language, speech, appearance and in every imaginable way we interact with each other. The way people demonstrate their innate sexuality varies according to their stage of life. It is expressed in family intimacy and as part of play in childhood, more overtly in adolescence and in physical sexual activity throughout adult life. However, as already mentioned, people in their later years are not seen by society as having sexual needs or the capacity for sexual expression. Those with physical and intellectual disabilities are also often viewed in the same way. People can, however, be very sexual without engaging in the complete act of intercourse. Touching, caressing, kissing, cuddling and so forth are all fundamental modes of sexual expression, and become even more important for people with increasing age, or for people who have physical limitations.

There is a prevailing misconception that women's sexuality declines with increasing age, and that older women who continue to engage in intercourse mostly do so to please their partner. Perpetuation of such myths is unhealthy and, if anything, results in many older women feeling uncomfortable about their ongoing sexuality. All women retain their capacity for sexual expression until death. Sexual activity might lessen with ageing in terms of coital frequency, but women do not suddenly stop being female when they reach a critical age and start dressing and acting like eunuchs! Innate sexuality endures, it is merely the mode of expression which changes.

How individual sexuality is manifested is influenced by the cultural and social environment, personal knowledge, past experiences and current expectations, physical and psychological well-being and, most importantly, the availability of a partner.

So, it is undeniable that human sexuality is innate and through life influences most aspects of our behaviour. Many mothers in recent years have been determined to avoid sexual stereotyping in their offspring so that their children can grow up free from the constraints of society's gender expectations. However, intrinsic sexuality dominates environmental influences. Children automatically discover their own sexuality, which persists inextricably from their sense of self.

As little girls grow up and pass through puberty into adult life their sexuality becomes more rigidly and culturally defined. Sexual identity and femininity easily become confused with social expectations in terms of partnerships and childbearing. Society dictates the modes in which sexuality can be acceptably expressed. There is obviously great variation in this according to peer group and community expectations. With few exceptions there is still the global assumption that women's sexuality is most acceptably manifest in a long-term, heterosexual relationship with childbearing and home-making as the desired outcomes. Women who either by circumstance or choice do not follow this path are often viewed as being less womanly than others. Some women who are infertile describe a sense of loss of their femininity. This is particularly common among women with premature ovarian failure, that is who no longer have normal sex hormone production by their ovaries. Some of my patients tell me that they feel their male partners see them as less feminine and less sexual because of their reproductive failure. In cultures where sexuality and reproduction are viewed as markers of personal success and fulfilment, pressure is probably greatest. I have encountered too many young women who are childless for various reasons who feel tacitly sexually disenfranchised. A sad aspect of this is that women are most often the harshest judges of all, and I quote Janine O'Leary-Cobb who wrote that 'women impose horrendously negative judgements on each other and on themselves. They confuse the packaging with the contents and adopt false and cruel criteria, viewing sexuality as a quality to be granted, or taken away, rather than as always there.' (A Friend Indeed, A Friend Indeed Inc., Montreal, 1996). We even have clichés which echo our disapproval of older women who are youthful or sexually suggestive in their appearance. We talk of 'mutton dressed up as lamb', and generally feel women should 'age gracefully'. Many of my patients feel it is socially acceptable for older men openly to have relationships with or marry much younger women, whereas the reverse does not apply. If a wealthy woman marries a much younger man he must be 'after her money', but when a wealthy man weds a much younger women, she is giving him a new lease on life!

Women are as sexual as men, something most women do not even recognise. They express their femaleness and sexuality in loving, caring for and nurturing others, and by touching and comforting. Sexuality is usually measured by frequency of intercourse or orgasm because we don't know how to measure frequency of touching or caressing, which are such essential modes of sexual expression, especially in the early and later years of life.

So, accepting that women's sexuality is enduring, what do we know about changing sexuality with ageing? The decline in sex steroids at the time of menopause impacts to varying degrees on female sexuality. It cannot be emphasised enough that every woman's experience of the menopause is personal and individual and depends on her past and present circumstances in terms of culture, social and psychological factors and health. In general, after transiting the menopause women experience fewer sexual thoughts and fantasies, lessened vaginal lubrication with intercourse and less sexual satisfaction. Sex hormone levels, particularly blood levels of testosterone, are associated with coital frequency, with higher levels being linked to more frequent sex. For many women these changes are subtle and do not interfere with their overall sexual relationships. In fact, most women appear to have no significant change in their sex lives after menopause, although up to twenty per cent report menopause has a significant impact on their sexual activity. One of the greatest predictors of a woman having a satisfying sexual relationship or experiences after menopause is the quality of the sexual aspects of her life before menopause, with those most satisfied with this aspect of their life in the late premenopausal years least likely to report problems. The availability of an interested partner appears to be a critical factor for older women, who often attribute lessened sexual activity to impotence or illness in their partner.

SEXUALITY AND THE MENOPAUSE

At all stages of life sexual health is determined in multifarious ways. During the menopausal transition and beyond, many factors potentially impact on a woman's sense and expression of sexuality. Factors known to be predictive of reduced sexual interest at menopause include general reduction in well-being, co-existence of other physical symptoms, negative attitudes towards the menopause, dissatisfaction with work or unemployment and depression. Menopause is still commonly regarded as a negative life event, which until quite recently has been little discussed, and still too often in hushed tones.

Apart from the effects of psychological adjustments to the menopause, which vary greatly in nature and significance between women, the physical changes resulting from both ageing and declining oestrogen levels affect female sexuality at this time. Societal attitudes to physical changes are also important. The physical trappings of increasing age such as greying hair, wrinkles and drooping breasts engender negative social responses as the antipathy of the beauty of youth. Society needs ongoing education and cultural change so that each life stage is seen to have its own positive as well as negative effects.

PHYSICAL EFFECTS OF AGEING ON SEXUAL ACTIVITY

In addition to circulating oestrogen levels falling at menopause, the nervous system and vascular system also decline with age. Loss of fat and glandular tissue combined with lessened muscle tone and tissue elasticity makes the breasts and other body regions more drooping and flabby. The cervix, uterus and ovaries shrink, the vagina becomes dry and the lining tissue thinner, and the clitoris, which retains its sensitivity, decreases in size. Oestrogen loss causes much of the discomfort of intercourse that may occur with ageing, and oestrogen replacement, even oestrogen creams applied locally, will successfully reverse symptoms such as vaginal dryness and contact bleeding with intercourse. The duration of orgasm is reduced in women over 50 years of age. In some women, uterine contractions during orgasm may become spasmodic and painful instead of being rhythmic and pleasurable. Alternatively, the contractions may become so mild in older women that they are not sure whether they have achieved orgasm. Following orgasm, resolution to an unstimulated state is more rapid in older women. However, women of all ages are capable of experiencing multiple orgasms.

Fundamentally, age is no deterrent to good sex. The changes of ageing may require some accommodation by both partners, but adjustments can always be made to permit ongoing sexual activity.

The impact of illness on sexual activity in women is not often discussed. Physically, coitus is no more taxing than a vigorous walk. For a woman with a heart condition sexual activity is usually safe if she is able to climb a flight of stairs or walk briskly for ten to fifteen minutes without any distress.

Diabetes is a common cause of impotence in men, but does not appear to affect either sexual desire or performance in women. Urinary tract and vaginal infections, such as thrush, are more common in diabetics, so practices such as emptying the bladder before and soon after intercourse are important.

Medications prescribed for various diseases can potentially affect female sexual function, but unfortunately have been little studied in women, as opposed to the vast literature on drug-induced impotence in men. Women on medication who experience diminished sexual desire or responsiveness should discuss this issue with their doctor.

Ageing has different effects on the four phases of the female sexual response: desire, plateau, orgasm and resolution. Testosterone is known to be important for sexual desire in both women and men (see page 187). Beyond the hormonal requirements, sexual arousal is achieved through touching, kissing, clitoral stimulation and erotic fantasies. In older women touch sensation is diminished as is vascular responsiveness, therefore nipple erection and genital response and congestion is lessened. Vaginal secretions are reduced and longer time is required for adequate lubrication to occur. Although the clitoris becomes smaller with age, the response to stimulation remains intact, but it usually takes longer to achieve a sexual plateau.

Many older women do not have a partner or are in a partnership with a person who suffers ill health or sexual dysfunction. Masturbation is less well accepted by women than men, but is an important sexual outlet for many women. Early research suggests that up to 25 per cent of women over the age of 70 masturbate. Mutual masturbation is a common, healthy, sexual practice for many couples when ill health prevents vaginal intercourse.

It is important that society frees older people from sexual taboos and misconceptions. Physical changes naturally occur with ageing, but mutual caring and adaptation to changing circumstances will enable an ongoing satisfactory sexual relationship. It is rare that the physiological changes of ageing warrant cessation of sexual activity. The low level of sexual desire unfortunately expressed by so many older women often strongly reflects negative societal feedback on ageing in general and sexual repression of older women specifically. Improving our attitudes towards ageing, increasing respect for older women in the community and liberalising our views on sexual expression in older people will hopefully free older women from imposed community constraints. Women with concerns about their sexual life should find a doctor or counsellor with whom they feel comfortable discussing this very personal but important aspect of their life. Sexual health is a significant component of overall health and well-being.

ANDROGENS IN WOMEN

Androgens are traditionally viewed as 'male' hormones, and in the case of women are usually only considered when there is concern about a woman having too many androgens, for example if she has excessive hairiness and acne. But androgens are sex hormones of major physiological significance in women, important for maintaining strong muscles and bones, positive protein balance, sexual desire and general well-being. Women who suffer androgen insufficiency experience a variety of physical and psychological symptoms which affect their quality of life. These include fatigue, depression, low libido, muscle weakness and bone loss.

What are androgens?

Androgens are sex hormones produced by both the ovaries and the adrenal glands in women and by the testes in men. They are known mostly for their masculinising effects in men namely, beard growth, deeper voice, balding, muscle strength and potency. The main androgens in women are the adrenal androgens and testosterone. Fifty per cent of female testosterone is produced by the ovaries and adrenal glands and released directly into the blood stream. The other 50 per cent comes from conversion of the adrenal androgens to testosterone in other parts of the body. Adrenal androgens are very important hormones as they are the main source of both testosterone and oestrogen after menopause. In fact, the level of one of the adrenal androgens known as *DHEA-S* in the blood stream is higher than that of any other human steroid, except cholesterol. One of the critical roles of androgens in women is oestrogen production. Oestrogen is an end product of androgen metabolism. The ovaries make oestrogen by converting testosterone to oestrogen. After menopause, when the ovaries no longer do this, female fat tissue is the main source of oestrogen, which is made by converting adrenal androgens to weaker oestrogens in the fat. Very little testosterone circulates freely in the blood stream. Instead 99 per cent of testosterone is bound tightly to a protein known as *sex hormone binding globulin* (SHBG). This is important when considering testosterone excess and testosterone deficiency. Factors which lower SHBG will result in more free testosterone circulating and therefore affected women are more likely to be masculinsed with hairiness or acne. In contrast, factors which increase SHBG will result in more testosterone being bound-up and less being free. Oestrogen therapy, either as the oral contraceptive pill or hormone replacement therapy, increases SHBG, resulting in reduced free testosterone and may cause lessened sexual desire and libido as a side effect.

Testosterone levels vary during the menstrual cycle just like other sex hormones, peaking during the middle phase of the menstrual cycle around the time of ovulation. Some believe this may be an in-built stimulus to increased sexual activity in women close to ovulation and nature's way of enhancing sexual activity at this time, thereby increasing the likelihood of conception. The oral contraceptive pill suppresses this midcycle increase in testosterone and may cause lessening of libido in some women.

Changes in androgens with ageing

Ageing affects female androgen production by two different mechanisms. Firstly, the adrenal glands produce progressively less androgens, specifically less DHEA, which are important sources of oestrogen and testosterone in elderly men and women. Why this happens is not known, nor are the specific effects of the decline in DHEA well understood. There is, however, increasing interest in DHEA as an anti-ageing therapy, as we will discuss. Secondly the menopause results in lessened ovarian androgen production, although this statement is somewhat controversial. The combined impact of ovarian failure at menopause and declining adrenal androgen production with age is that older women have less testosterone circulating than young women. In the past, few people were interested in this change, as already discussed, as it has been socially acceptable for older women to be less sexual. Awareness of the importance of androgens has been evoked not only by interested clinicians and researchers but also by young women with androgen deficiency from either surgical removal of their ovaries or premature menopause, and the vocal baby-boomer lobby who continue to demand quality of life.

Unlike oestrogen which falls precipitously at menopause, testosterone levels in women decline gradually so that women in their forties have blood testosterone levels which are on average half of those of women in their twenties. The testosterone level of a 45-year-old woman complaining of low libido may well be in the 'normal range' for the test, but still be much lower than what she has been used to in the past. Such a woman may well benefit in terms of her libido and well-being by subtle testosterone replacement, still maintaining her levels in the 'normal range', rather than by psychological treatment or anti-depressant therapy.

Women who have their ovaries surgically removed are subject to a sudden drop in blood testosterone levels and frequently experience ongoing symptoms, despite supposedly adequate hormone replacement therapy with oestrogen. Common symptoms include impaired sexual desire and function, lessened well-being, loss of energy, depression and measurable loss of bone. As the absolute blood level of testosterone begins to decline in the decade preceding menopause it is not surprising that many women experience similar symptoms in their premenopausal years. The cause of these symptoms is rarely recognised or understood, and virtually never treated.

Androgens and post-menopausal sexuality

There are significant associations between menopausal status and declining sexual activity and coital frequency. When women have been studied from their premenopausal through to their post-menopausal years, specific patterns have been observed. Mean weekly rates of sexual intercourse declined over the menopausal transition period. Compared with pre-menopause, the women after menopause had significantly fewer sexual thoughts or fantasies, experienced increased lack of vaginal lubrication during sex and were less satisfied with their partners as lovers. These changes were closely correlated with the decline in both oestrogen and testosterone with menopause, although the fall in testosterone was most strongly associated with lessened coital frequency. Clearly, declining health and sexual interest as well as availability of a partner impacts on coital frequency, but this was not a significant factor in this study.

Furthermore, it has been suggested that lessened sexuality after menopause may be a self-fulfilling prophecy for some women. However, the effect of anticipation of change in sexuality in women entering menopause has also been looked at, and the association between expectation of less sex and what is actually experienced is very weak.

In summary, there is increasing agreement that androgens play a key role in human female sexuality and that androgen deprivation after menopause contributes to a reduced sexual desire and responsiveness in a number of women. This aspect of adult female reproductive health is too often trivialised. Young women who suffer either premature menopause or who undergo surgical removal of both ovaries early in life commonly experience great distress from their loss of libido. It impinges on their intimate relationships and potential to develop new, satisfactory, sexual relationships and as one young women has said, results not only in loss of femininity, but of sexual 'personhood'. Such women are usually very responsive to testosterone replacement therapy, and the significance of restoring sexuality to these women must not be undervalued.

Androgen replacement therapy

Oestrogen replacement at menopause eliminates or lessens hot flushes, reverses vaginal dryness, and hence improves lubrication with intercourse, and improves general well-being, but has little effect on libido. In contrast, androgen replacement using different formulations of testosterone appears to enhance various parameters of sexual motivation including intensity of sexual drive, arousal and frequency of sexual fantasies not induced by oestrogen replacement alone. Testosterone replacement therapy for women does not have widespread acceptance, particularly in North America, but is increasingly becoming more available as women demand acknowledgment of this aspect of their lives.

Testosterone replacement for women is available in the form of testosterone implants and injections. No form of oral testosterone has been designed for or approved for use in women in Australia, although oral testosterone is available in the US. Testosterone injections used for androgen replacement in men are sometimes given to women, but there have been no studies addressing the use of this form of treatment in women and little is known about the suitable dosage, safety or efficacy of testosterone-only injections in this context. An injectable form of testosterone combined with oestrogen is available but little used as it must be given frequently, and many women find this alternative both uncomfortable and inconvenient.

Testosterone implants at present seem to be the best option for androgen replacement in women. They are approved for this purpose in the UK and parts of Europe and, although not officially approved for this indication in Australia, they are in common usage. There is a body of scientific data demonstrating the short-term (up to two years) safety of testosterone implants, but no longer-term studies have yet been done. Usually they are inserted under the skin in the lower abdomen using a simple procedure, with or without the oestrogen implants that are used by many women as an alternative mode of oestrogen replacement therapy. Oestrogen implants are approved for use by women in Australia. When combined with oestrogen implants, testosterone implant therapy has been shown to significantly enhance sexual activity, satisfaction, pleasure, fantasy and orgasm in post-menopausal women. It has been suggested that these observed effects of testosterone replacement occur because testosterone is converted to oestrogen in the brain and then the increased level of brain oestrogen induces these changes. However, women treated with oestrogen alone do not experience the same sexual enhancement as those given combined oestrogen and testosterone therapy and the beneficial effects appear to be specifically due to the testosterone.

There are several important points to note regarding testosterone replacement therapy.

- Testosterone replacement therapy should not be given to post-menopausal women without oestrogen replacement simultaneously.
- When administered by testosterone implants or injections, blood testosterone levels should be measured at regular intervals to prevent overdosing and development of undesirable, masculinising side effects.
- Published studies have shown short-term safety and efficacy of testosterone replacement by implants in women. There is little published addressing safety, dosage or efficacy of oral (tablet) testosterone replacement (other than *methyltestosterone*) in women and, until such time, this form of testosterone replacement cannot be recommended. Although oral methyltestosterone is still available in North America, it cannot be prescribed in Australia. Methyltestosterone taken orally can have undesirable effects on the liver and its use is not recommended.
- Testosterone implants used for testosterone replacement in women do not adversely affect blood cholesterol levels when administered with oestrogen. Without oestrogen replacement, however, testosterone therapy could potentially negatively affect blood cholesterol levels.
- Cosmetic side effects of testosterone therapy are extremely rare when blood levels are kept in the normal range for

women, hence monitoring with blood tests during treatment is essential. Potential masculinising effects include the development of acne, increased body hair, balding and deepening of the voice. Testosterone replacement therefore should not be used by women who suffer from any of these conditions.

- There is no available information regarding the influence of testosterone replacement on breast cancer development. Certainly, there is no evidence to date that testosterone replacement via implants affects breast cancer occurrence.
- Testosterone treatment does not make women gain weight. Post-menopausal women treated with oestrogen and testosterone implants usually experience a modest increase in muscle bulk, a reduction in total body fat, but no change in overall body weight.

Androgens and bone loss after menopause

Androgenic hormones are known to be important in the maintenance of bone mass in both men and women. Even before menopause, bone mass in women is associated with blood testosterone levels, with greater bone mass observed in women with higher levels of circulating free testosterone. Androgens stimulate bone cell activity and hence bone formation. In contrast, oestrogen inhibits the cells which breakdown bone and thus blocks bone reabsorption. Therefore, after menopause, oestrogen replacement therapy prevents loss of bone by blocking the activity of bone reabsorbing cells. There is strong evidence that testosterone replacement after menopause enhances bone formation and in combination with oestrogen actually increases bone mass. At this time, low bone density is not an indication for testosterone treatment. However, testosterone replacement appears potentially to play an important therapeutic role in the prevention and treatment of post-menopausal bone loss which warrants further investigation.

Adrenal androgens in women

As outlined earlier, the adrenal glands are vital sources of sex hormones for both men and women. These glands are quiescent during early childhood but 'switch on' and begin to produce sufficient androgens in prepubertal boys and girls to induce the first changes of puberty known as *adrenarche*. The triggers for this are unknown. This increase in adrenal hormones induces sexual hair growth, increased oiliness of the skin and scalp and adult body odour, and paves the way for sexual maturation. Although from the mid-thirties on, circulating levels of the adrenal hormone DHEA decline linearly with age in both men and women, it is the main natural sex hormone produced in the body of women after menopause. It is converted in body tissues to both oestrogen and testosterone, although it is unclear as to which of these latter hormones is mostly responsible for the biological effects of DHEA. Its effects are probably mediated through both. DHEA has also been hailed as a possible anti-ageing drug, reinstating the essence of youth. Replacement therapy with DHEA to women with advancing age results in restoration of androgen levels, including testosterone and DHEA itself, to premenopausal levels. It has been reported that DHEA therapy results in enhanced well-being and increased energy with varying effects on libido. Preliminary evidence indicates DHEA may protect against bone loss after menopause, or even result in increased bone formation, but this requires further evaluation and documentation. Multiple other biological effects have been attributed to DHEA therapy, including anti-cancer actions and immune system stimulation, alongside claims that it can be used to treat illnesses such as chronic fatigue syndrome. At this point, the therapeutic role of DHEA remains both unclear and controversial. There have been some concerns about its toxic effects in humans and it should not be taken outside the confines of a properly conducted and monitored research study.

SUMMING UP

Androgens are important hormones in women, having diverse biological actions throughout life. The decline in androgen production by both the adrenal glands and the ovaries which begins a decade before the average age of naturally occurring menopause, has significant impact on the physical, psychological and sexual well-being of women. The clinical repercussions of androgen insufficiency in women have only recently been recognised and, although still controversial in some countries, testosterone replacement therapy for symptomatic women is becoming an increasingly available option. Unfortunately, treatment is limited by the lack of user-friendly testosterone formulations, but the development of a testosterone patch for women is highly likely in the near future.

Side effects of testosterone replacement are a concern for doctors inexperienced in androgen replacement in women. Genuine side effects are, in fact, rare when a replacement regimen is instituted by a physician familiar with this form of therapy and when women are properly monitored. However, testosterone implants should only be administered by a physician experienced in the procedure and the effects of this therapy, and only with concurrent oestrogen replacement.

The option of testosterone replacement is important for all post-menopausal women but is particularly so for young women who should be at their prime in terms of sexuality but who are robbed of this celebration of life by either premature or surgically induced menopause.

THE AIM OF PREVENTIVE HEALTH CARE

Every woman is biologically different and uniquely influenced by her social and cultural environment, life experiences and education. Thus, the health needs for various women differ throughout life in accordance with differing individual physical needs and personal expectations.

Health for women is broader than reproductive health, and the ultimate aim should be to enable physical, psychological and emotional well-being. Clearly, there are specific disease states, such as gynaecological conditions, which only affect women. However, several conditions including osteoporosis, Alzheimer's disease, depression, eating disorders and obesity disproportionately affect women more than men. I have described how patterns of illness in women often differ from those observed in men, and that knowledge from research studies involving mostly or only men cannot always be directly translated to women. More research is needed to expand our understanding of certain conditions in women such as heart disease, diabetes and stroke. This is essential for the development of appropriate prevention and treatment strategies for women.

Women continue to be the main health and lifestyle educators for the family unit. Hence health education for women translates directly into education for their children, partners, parents or, put more embracingly, into education for the community. Through education and awareness, it is possible for women to take command of their health and make responsible health choices. Consequent to improving health and nutrition, people are living longer and, globally, we are an ageing population. However, the greater life expectancy of women than men is associated with many years of disability due to ill health. The average Australian woman is likely to experience fourteen years of physical handicap in her later life, of which an average of six years is of severe handicap due to ill health. Not only is this a burden to the community in terms of monetary costs, but the human costs in terms of loss of quality of life in old age are unacceptable. We have come to not only associate ageing with declining health, physical dependence and social isolation, but more and more to accept these as inevitable. I believe that much of the ill health which affects people in later years can be prevented by having a healthy lifestyle throughout life. Healthy living and preventive health should begin in childhood. Investment in our own health by being informed and positively 'living well' is the wisest insurance policy to which we can contribute.

Preventive health measures can only be successful if people are given the opportunity to learn about their bodies and health needs, and the impact of lifestyle factors on health. Knowledge alone, however, is not enough. We must be responsible for our own health. This responsibility ranges from choosing whether or not to smoke cigarettes or drink alcohol, through to the types and quantities of food eaten, physical exercise and recognising and dealing with stress.

It also means being responsible users of health facilities. This means actively interacting with the doctor or health carer, knowing the name of any diagnosis that is made, asking about tests and treatments and why they are needed, and making optimal health decisions in conjunction with the treating doctor.

Women should seek out a family physician with whom they relate comfortably and feel they can discuss any health issues of concern. It is important to try to be objective. For example, there is the prevailing attitude that everything labelled 'natural' is healthy and can do no harm, whereas traditional Western medicines are viewed as drugs with the potential to cause harm. Myths such as these can result in people denying themselves sensible, appropriate health care. It is difficult to sort out the barrage of mixed health information with which we are being confronted. Question the sources of any new health recommendations and try to ascertain whether the information presented is someone's personal belief or established fact. Much of what is written or said is influenced by biases. Again, information about the natural therapies is a good example. The information presented is too often overly influenced by the limited knowledge, beliefs and (lack of) objectivity of the source.

The roles of women in society are less rigidly defined today than in past decades, and different women have varying health needs and should make health choices appropriate to their own lifestyle. However, women generally pack more into their lives today than ever before. Life is increasingly pressured and this can cause both physical and psychological stress, and generate relationship stresses. There is a tendency for women to continually 'put in', and feel uncomfortable about taking time for themselves. Everyone needs some personal space, both in the physical sense and also as mind space. We all need some personal time to switch off or indulge ourselves, and for some women this may be as simple as making time to sit and read the newspaper. Everyone needs a break from their immediate environment to be alone to reflect.

We shouldn't feel guilty or selfish about making time for ourselves. Time out, or personal space, is stress-relieving and regenerating and helps us cope better with each other and life's demands. It is important to prioritise your life and set aside the time to find time that is your own. I believe that this is an important part of women being responsible for themselves and for their own well-being.

There are so many choices to be made in life. For the individual it ultimately comes down to personal expectations in terms of quality of life and short- and long-term goals. I believe that quality of life is paramount and that life is precious. Don't let it slip by. Be well and enjoy every moment.

Osteoporosis   Loss of bone from the skeleton to the extent that bones are at high risk of fracture.

Ovulation   Release of a mature egg from the ovary into the fallopian tube.

Phytoestrogen   Plant chemicals with oestrogen-like actions.

Phytomedicines   Plant medicines.

Pituitary   A small gland situated under the centre of the brain which produces hormones which stimulate the other major hormone producing glands in the body. Also acts as the link between the brain and the body's hormonal systems.

Placebo   An inactive tablet given as a 'dummy' tablet in research studies.

Polycystic ovary syndrome (PCO)   A state in which the ovaries contain multiple minicysts. Often linked to excessive body hair, obesity and diabetes.

Premature menopause   Menopause before the age of 40.

Premenstrual syndrome (PMS)   A cluster of symptoms which recur in the days before each menstruation.

Primary amenorrhoea   The state of never having menstruated.

Progesterone   The female hormone made by the ovaries, especially following ovulation.

Prolactin   Produced by the pituitary and stimulates breast milk production.

Prostaglandins   Chemicals produced by the body which may cause various biological effects including the pain of menstruation.

Resorcylic acid lactone   Chemical with oestrogen activity found in fungus, not true phytoestrogen.

Saturated fat   Fats derived from animal products such as meat and dairy products.

Secondary amenorrhoea   Cessation of menstruation in a woman who has previously menstruated.

Systolic pressure   The upper figure recorded when blood pressure is measured.

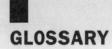

GLOSSARY

Adrenal androgens   Hormones produced by the adrenal glands which have testosterone-like actions or which can be metabolised to testosterone.

Adrenal stimulating hormone (ACTH)   Produced by the pituitary and stimulates adrenal gland function.

Amenorrhoea   Absence of menstruation.

Androgens   Hormones in both men and women which are important for muscle strength, bone formation and growth of sexual hair. Higher levels of androgens in men result in the features of masculinity.

Angina   Pain arising from insufficient blood flow to the heart muscle.

Angioplasty   A medical procedure in which a narrowed artery is opened up by the inflation of a small balloon which has been fed into the narrowed segment.

Anorexia nervosa   An illness featuring extreme weight loss, disturbed body image and a fear of being overweight.

Atherosclerosis   Hardening and narrowing of arteries by cholesterol and fat deposits.

Body mass index (BMI)   A formula for correcting body weight for height so that body weights can be compared. It is calculated by dividing body weight in kilograms by the square of the height in metres.

Bulimia   An eating disorder characterised by binge-eating, vomiting and laxative abuse associated with shame and low self-esteem.

Cardiovascular disease   Disease of the heart and/or blood vessels.

Cholesterol An essential compound for human cell structure and also for the production of important hormones. When cholesterol levels in the blood are increased, there is a heightened risk of atherosclerosis.

Congenital adrenal hyperplasia An hereditary condition characterised by abnormal production of hormones by the adrenal glands.

Coronary artery disease Disease of the main arteries to the heart usually caused by cholesterol build-up and restriction of blood flow through these arteries.

Coumestrol A class of plant oestrogen.

Diabetes mellitus Also known as *sugar diabetes*. A disease in which the body is either unable to make adequate insulin or becomes insensitive to insulin and blood glucose levels are increased.

Diastolic pressure The lower figure recorded when blood pressure is measured.

Dysmenorrhoea Painful menstruation.

Dysplasia Presence of abnormal cells.

Endocrinologist A physician who specialises in the action of hormones and the treatment of hormonal disorders.

Endometrium The lining tissue of the uterus which is lost during menstruation.

Fatty streaks Yellow streaks in arteries which are early signs of cholesterol and fat being deposited.

Follicle stimulating hormone (FSH) Produced by the pituitary and stimulates the ovaries (and the testes in men).

Follicles Nests of cells in the ovary which contain a developing egg.

High density (HDL) cholesterol The form of cholesterol which is important in the clearance of cholesterol from the blood and tissues back to the liver. High levels are associated with lower risk of atherosclerosis.

Hirsutism Having 'excessive' facial and/or body hair.

Hypertension High blood pressure.

Hysterectomy Surgical removal of the uterus.

Insulin resistance When the body becomes less sensitiv to insulin and higher blood levels are needed for a 'no mal' effect.

Isoflavone A class of plant oestrogen.

Leptin A protein found in the blood that appears to affe food intake and levels of activity in humans and anima

Lignan A class of plant oestrogen.

Lipids A general collective term for the various types blood cholesterol and fats.

Low density (LDL) cholesterol The form of cholest which circulates in the blood and is taken up by the lir cells of the arteries causing atherosclerosis.

Luteal phase The part of the menstrual cycle that s after ovulation and ends with menstruation, during w time progesterone levels rise.

Luteinising hormone (LH) Produced by the pituitary stimulates the ovaries. It is the prime stimulus for lation.

Menarche The first menstrual period.

Menopause The last natural menstrual period. Repr the end of a woman's reproductive phase.

Menstrual migraine Migraine headaches occurring larly at the time of menstruation.

Myocardial infarction Commonly known as a heart This occurs when an artery to the heart becomes c narrowed or blocked and an area of heart muscle

Non-steroidal anti-inflammatory drugs (NSAIDs) ications which have an anti-inflammation action.

Obesity Having excessive body weight to a degree is associated with significant health risks. Usually ered to be a body mass index greater than 30 k

Oestrogen The major female hormone, produced nantly by the ovaries.

Oophorectomy Surgical removal of an ovary.

Testosterone The main circulating androgen (hormone causing male characteristics) in men and women.

Thrombolysis therapy Specialised treatment given to break down a newly formed clot in a blood vessel.

Trans fat Artificial fats present in manufactured foods which have been linked to coronary artery disease.

Triglycerides Blood fats which circulate in the blood.

INDEX

abdominal bloating 38
abdominal fat 164, 165, 166, 167, 171
abdominal hair 58
abdominal ultrasound 64, 115
Aboriginal people: Westernised lifestyle and 166–7
absinthe 91–2
acetazolamide 48
acne: androgens and 59; drug treatment for 66, 194; hirsutism and 59, 60, 61, 62, 63; SHBG and 189; testosterone therapy and 194
ACTH 63, 201
Addison's disease 109, 110
adolescents: breast cancer prevention and 144; diet and 153; eating disorders in 22; growth spurts of 26; hormone treatments for 55, 118–19; menstrual disorders in 31–3, 55, 144; obesity in 19–21, 144, 153, 154; PMS and 40; POF and 62, 113, 118–19; sexuality and 11; *see also* athletes; children; gymnasts; puberty
adrenal androgens 59, 65, 188, 189, 195, 201
adrenal gland disease 109, 110, 115
adrenal hormones 41, 53, 59, 60, 65, 187–95, 196
adrenaline 59
adrenarche 195
age and ageing: androgen changes and 189–90, 195; attitudes to 13–14, 198; body hair and 60; oestrogen and 2, 170; positive aspects of 13–14; sexuality and 181–2, 183–4, 190–1; weight gains and 163, 164, 167, 171, 172; *see also* menopause and menopausal symptoms
alcohol: breast cancer and 128, 129, 130, 136, 137, 143; eating disorders and 23; ill health and 8; menstrual disorders and 34, 46
alcoholic extracts 87
Aldactone 66
alfalfa 73, 86, 87–8
Alzheimer's disease 197
amenorrhoea 31–2, 62, 64, 66, 113, 114, 165, 201
American ginseng 89

Androcur 66–7
androgens: bone loss and 194; breast cancer and 126; herbs with activities like 93–4; hirsutism and 59–60, 61, 62, 63, 64, 65; oestrogen and 188–9; overview of 188–9; ovulation and 29, 165, 189; POF and 111–12, 119; replacement therapy for 191–4; women and 187–95, 196
angina 148, 150, 159, 173, 201
angioplasty 175, 201
anorexia nervosa 9, 14, 21, 22–5, 114, 201
anti-androgen therapy 63, 65, 66–7
anti-inflammatory agents 35, 46
anti-oestrogens 71, 78, 141
antioxidants 132, 148, 171, 175–7
anti-prostaglandin therapy 35, 36, 46
aphrodisiacs 93–4
arthritis and obesity 21
Asia: attitudes to ageing in 14; BMI in 167–8; breast cancer in 135; incidence of diseases in 70, 77, 78, 135, 168; menopausal symptoms in 74, 75, 76; obesity in 15–16, 168; phytoestrogens and diet in 70, 77, 78, 94; *see also* Oriental ginseng
aspirin 82, 83, 145, 148, 150, 179, 180
atherosclerosis 15, 21, 101, 149–51, 153, 158, 162, 163, 164, 165, 171, 173, 177, 201
atherosclerotic plaques 149, 150
athletes: bone loss and 49; eating disorders in 25; hormone levels and 48, 49, 50–1, 52, 53, 54, 55; menstrual problems and 48–53, 54; reproductive problems and 48–53, 54, 113, 144; stress and 5, 50, 51
atopic eczema 92
Australia: body hair attitudes in 56, 57; body weight of children from 19–20, 153; cancer and 4, 122–3,138, 139; consumption of saturated fats in 160; diet of children in 20; heart disease in 151, 152; *see also* Aboriginal people
autoimmune diseases and POF 103, 109–10, 115